WHITE WINE
DIET

THE
WHITE WINE
DIET
LOSE ALL THE WEIGHT YOU WANT,
WITHOUT FEELING DEPRIVED

CARLY NEWMAN

metro

Published by Metro Publishing Ltd,
3, Bramber Court, 2 Bramber Road,
London W14 9PB, England

www.blake.co.uk

First published in paperback in 2004

ISBN 1 84358 084 5

British Library Cataloguing-in-Publication Data:

A catalogue record for this book is available
from the British Library.

Design by www.envydesign.co.uk

Printed in Great Britain by Bookmarque

1 3 5 7 9 10 8 6 4 2

Papers used by Metro Publishing are natural, recyclable products made
from wood grown in sustainable forests. The manufacturing processes
conform to the environmental regulations of the country of origin.

Contents

1
Why White Wine is Good For You

It sounds like a gimmick, doesn't it? After all, aren't we always told of the health risks of drinking too much alcohol? And doesn't it make you fat?

Well, too much alcohol *is* bad for you. And yes, too much does make you fat. I want to make it perfectly clear at the outset of this book that, if you over-drink, then both your health and your waistline will suffer.

But healthy eating, and sensible, effective dieting, is all about moderation – a principle that is at the heart of this book. If you love wine, then there is no reason why it should not be part of a good diet. And, indeed, there are many positive reasons why you *should* treat yourself to a chilled glass of delicious, crisp white wine – or even two! To find out why, read on …

Have you ever heard of the 'French paradox'? It's a phrase scientists use to explain their observation that, although the French traditionally have a diet that is heavy in all sorts of high-fat foods – cream, butter, red meat – they have a much lower rate of heart disease than those in other countries who eat seemingly more healthily.

The reason, scientists discovered, was because the French tipple of choice was wine. They found that substances in wine are very effective in lowering our cholesterol count and essentially 'cleaning' the arteries: so the bad work being done by all the cream and butter was being undone by the wine.

Now don't get your hopes up. This isn't an excuse to go on a cream-cake and wine binge! The point I am making is that this is just one of the positive effects of drinking wine in moderation. There are many others:

WINE AND CANCER

Research has indicated that wine, in moderation, is effective in helping people avoid and fight cancer. It contains a cancer-suppressing chemical called resveratrol. It is also high in antioxidants, which are extremely effective in the fight against the disease.

WINE AND STROKES

Scientists have discovered that the alcohol found in wine breaks up blood clots and increases the level of good cholesterol in the blood. This keeps the arteries from clogging up, and so helps prevent the common stroke.

WINE AND ULCERS

Ulcer infections are caused by a bacterium called *helico bacterpylori*. Scientists conducted a study of 1800 people and discovered that, compared with non-drinkers, those who had one glass of wine a day had 7% fewer of these bacteria; those who had two glasses of wine a day had 18% fewer; and those who drank three glasses of wine a day had 33% fewer.

WINE AND BRAIN DISORDERS

Scientists have learned that that magic chemical resveratrol (the one that helps fight cancer) helps the brain regenerate its cells, so avoiding brain disorders. There is no proof that it prevents conditions such as Alzheimer's and Parkinson's, but scientists are currently investigating that possibility.

WINE AND THE LUNGS

Wine – and especially white wine – seems to have a long-term positive effect on the health of the lungs. It is thought that this is because wine contains a high level of the antioxidant molecules called flavonoids.

So there you have it. Far from being bad for you, a small amount of wine each day can actually have positive health benefits.

2
How Does the White Wine Diet Work?

So how does wine fit in with a weight-loss plan? Surely the first rule of a diet is to cut out the alcohol?

Well, that's not necessarily the case. As with any good diet, the secret lies in portion control. One glass of white wine contains, on average, 85 calories – 110 if it's sparkling. (See the list on page 9 for the exact calorie contents of different types of wine.)

What we're going to do is work out what your calorie intake should be in order for you to start losing weight safely and effectively. Once we've done this, we can design a tailor-made eating plan that contains just the right number of calories – and we will build two glasses of wine a day into this eating plan.

This book contains all the information you'll need to help you do this, including:

1. Calorie intake tables for both men and women (pages 13-18)

2. Loads of delicious, carefully constructed recipes with precise calorie contents so that you can design your own meal plans and eat tasty, easy food while shedding the pounds

3. Some sample meal plans for various different calorie intakes

4. An invaluable list of foods and their calorie contents

5. A list of essential tips for cooking food in a healthy, low-fat way – vital whether you're following the white wine diet or not

HOW DO I START THE DIET?

Easy. Go to the calorie intake tables on pages 13-18 and work out how many calories you ought to be eating *if you're not on a diet*, according to your sex, age, current weight and lifestyle.

For example, if you are a 45-year-old woman with a sedentary job – working at a desk in an office perhaps – and you currently weigh 11 stone, your recommended daily calorie intake is 2140. That means that, if you consume 2140 calories a day, you will stay the same weight. If you consume more calories, you will gain weight; and if you consume fewer calories, you will lose weight.

All you need to do now is a simple sum. Subtract 700 calories from your recommended calorie intake, which will make your body find the extra calories it needs from your fat reserves, so making you lose weight. You are also going to allow yourself two 120ml glasses of wine per day, so knock off another 180 calories from your intake. (Note that this depends on what sort of white wine you are drinking – see page 9).

I also recommend that you drink half a pint of skimmed milk every day. This contains 100 calories, so subtract this from your calorie intake too.

This will give you a calorie intake of 1160 – including your two glasses of white wine. *If you've worked out your recommended daily calorie intake correctly, then by reducing it in this way you WILL lose weight. There's no question about it.*

Now go to the recipes. Choose breakfasts, lunches and dinners that add up to your desired calorie intake. If you want a bit of help, look at the weekly menu plans, and if you need to add extra calories, do so from the list of foods and their calories on pages 191-198.

It really is as simple as that. In a nutshell:

- Work out your daily recommended calorie intake from the tables on pages 13-18
- Subtract 700 calories
- Subtract 100 calories for half a pint of skimmed milk every day
- Subtract the number of calories in two glasses of your favourite white wine (see the list on page 9)
- Now you've got your final White Wine Diet calorie intake, choose from the delicious dieters' recipes (see pages 23-174)

Why not use the table below to work out how many calories you should consume in order to drink wine and lose weight:

Recommended calorie intake   _____
(From the tables on pages 12-17)

minus

Number of calories in a glass of
your chosen white wine _____
(See the list on page 9)

                           x 2 _____

minus

Number of calories in half a pint of
skimmed milk   100

minus

Number of calories to subtract for
weight loss   700

equals

Target calorie intake for the
white wine diet   _____

(i.e. How many calories you can consume and still drink half a pint of milk and two glasses of delicious white wine every day)

HOW MANY CALORIES ARE THERE IN A GLASS OF WHITE WINE?

Wine contains no fat, but it does have calories because of the alcohol and sugar content. It is possible to work out the exact calorie content of a 120ml glass of wine by using the formula: 6.4 x alcohol percentage of the wine. But that is rather hard work, so broadly speaking, the sweeter a wine, the higher the calorie content. For example, a 120ml glass of dry Chablis contains about 85 calories, whereas the same measure of sweet Sauternes contains 115 calories.

It is not easy to give an exact calorie count for all the different wines you are likely to encounter. *However, for the purposes of the White Wine Diet, use the following list and you won't go wrong:*

Dry white wine: 85 calories
Medium white wine: 90 calories
Champagne/sparkling wine: 105 calories
Sweet/dessert wines: 115 calories

Remember to take into account which type of wine you are drinking when you work out what your calorie intake should be on the White Wine Diet!

On the White Wine Diet, you are allowed two 120ml glasses a day – but, if you prefer a longer drink, why not make a spritzer with half wine and half mineral water. You are allowed four of these a day.

3
The Calorie Intake Tables

On the following pages you will find lists of the recommended calorie intakes for men and women of different ages. These represent the number of calories you need to consume if you are to maintain your current weight.

The tables are divided into the following groups:

Women aged 18–29
Women aged 30–59
Women aged over 60
Men aged 18–29
Men aged 30–59
Men aged over 60

Go to the correct table for your sex and age group. You then need to decide if you are sedentary, active or very active. If you drive to work and sit at a desk all day, you are sedentary. If you do a moderate amount of exercise – perhaps you walk to work, or go swimming a few times a week – then you are active. If you do vigorous exercise for more than half an hour every day, you are very active. Be honest with yourself. You can then work out the recommended calorie intake for a person of your weight.

By going to the table in chapter two, you can then work out how many calories you should be consuming on the White Wine Diet.

The Calorie Intake Tables

Daily calorie requirements of women aged 18–29			
Weight (stone)*	Total number of calories required		
	Sedentary	Active	Very Active
7	1720	1950	2180
7.5	1790	2030	2270
8	1860	2110	2360
8.5	1930	2190	2450
9	2000	2270	2540
9.5	2070	2350	2630
10	2140	2430	2710
10.5	2210	2510	2800
11	2280	2590	2890
11.5	2360	2670	2980
12	2430	2750	3070
12.5	2500	2830	3160
13	2570	2830	3160
13.5	2640	2990	3340
14	2710	3070	3430
14.5	2780	3150	3520
15	2850	3230	3610
15.5	2918	3306	3696
16	2998	3386	3785
16.5	3060	3468	3876
17	3130	3548	3965
17.5	3200	3628	4053
18	3270	3706	4142
18.5	3342	3788	4233
19	3411	3866	4321
19.5	3480	3944	4408
20	3555	4029	4503

*1 stone = 6.35kg

Daily calorie requirements of women aged 30–59

Weight (stone)*	Total number of calories required		
	Sedentary	Active	Very Active
7	1820	2070	2310
7.5	1860	2110	2360
8	1900	2160	2410
8.5	1940	2200	2460
9	1980	2250	2510
9.5	2020	2290	2560
10	2060	2340	2610
10.5	2100	2380	2660
11	2140	2430	2710
11.5	2180	2470	2760
12	2220	2520	2810
12.5	2260	2560	2860
13	2300	2600	2910
13.5	2340	2650	2960
14	2380	2700	3010
14.5	2420	2740	3060
15	2460	2790	3110
15.5	2468	2796	3126
16	2506	2841	3175
16.5	2550	2890	3230
17	2584	2929	3274
17.5	2625	2975	3325
18	2661	3016	3371
18.5	2700	3060	3420
19	2738	3102	3468
19.5	2778	3148	3519
20	2820	3196	3572

*1 stone = 6.35kg

The Calorie Intake Tables

Weight	Total number of calories required		
(stone)*	Sedentary	Active	Very Active
7	1500	1700	1900
7.5	1542	1750	1950
8	1590	1800	2010
8.5	1630	1850	2070
9	1670	1900	2120
9.5	1720	1950	2180
10	1760	2000	2230
10.5	1810	2050	2290
11	1850	2100	2340
11.5	1890	2150	2400
12	1940	2200	2450
12.5	1980	2240	2510
13	2030	2300	2570
13.5	2070	2350	2620
14	2110	2400	2680
14.5	2160	2450	2730
15	2200	2500	2790
15.5	2328	2638	2949
16	2372	2688	3004
16.5	2415	2737	3059
17	2458	2786	3114
17.5	2500	2834	3167
18	2546	2885	3224
18.5	2589	2934	3279
19	2631	2982	3333
19.5	2674	3031	3388
20	2715	3077	3439

Daily calorie requirements of women aged over 60

*1 stone = 6.35kg

Daily calorie requirements of men aged 18–29

Weight (stone)*	Total number of calories required		
	Sedentary	Active	Very Active
8	2180	2480	2770
8.5	2260	2570	2870
9	2340	2650	2960
9.5	2410	2730	3050
10	2480	2810	3140
10.5	2550	2890	3230
11	2620	2970	3320
11.5	2700	3060	3410
12	2770	3140	3510
12.5	2840	3220	3600
13	2910	3300	3690
13.5	2980	3380	3780
14	3060	3460	3870
14.5	3130	3550	3960
15	3200	3630	4050
15.5	3270	3710	4140
16	3330	3770	4220
16.5	3420	3870	4330
17	3490	3950	4420
17.5	3548	4020	4494
18	3615	4097	4579
18.5	3690	4182	4674
19	3765	4267	4769
19.5	3832	4344	4854
20	3908	4428	4950

*1 stone = 6.35kg

The Calorie Intake Tables

Weight (stone)*	Total number of calories required		
	Sedentary	Active	Very Active
8	2190	2480	2770
8.5	2240	2540	2840
9	2300	2600	2910
9.5	2350	2670	2980
10	2410	2730	3050
10.5	2460	2790	3120
11	2520	2850	3190
11.5	2570	2920	3260
12	2630	2980	3330
12.5	2680	3040	3400
13	2740	3100	3470
13.5	2790	3160	3540
14	2850	3230	3640
14.5	2900	3290	3680
15	2960	3350	3750
15.5	3010	3410	3810
16	3060	3460	3870
16.5	3120	3540	2950
17	3180	3600	4020
17.5	3225	3655	4085
18	3276	3713	4150
18.5	3330	3774	4218
19	3390	3842	4294
19.5	3442	3902	4360
20	3495	3961	4427

Daily calorie requirements of men aged 30–59

*1 stone = 6.35kg

Daily calorie requirements of men aged over 60

Weight (stone)*	Total number of calories required		
	Sedentary	Active	Very Active
8	1773	2009	2246
8.5	1830	2074	2318
9	1884	2135	2386
9.5	1941	2200	2459
10	1996	2263	2529
10.5	2052	2326	2599
11	2109	2390	2671
11.5	2164	2453	2742
12	2220	2516	2812
12.5	2276	2579	2882
13	2332	2644	2954
13.5	2386	2705	3023
14	2444	2769	3095
14.5	2499	2832	3165
15	2556	2897	3238
15.5	2610	2958	3306
16	2666	3021	3376
16.5	2722	3086	3448
17	2778	3148	3519
17.5	2832	3210	3587
18	2889	3274	3659
18.5	2946	3339	3732
19	3000	3400	3800
19.5	3057	3465	3872
20	3112	3528	3942

*1 stone = 6.35kg

4

The Food-loving Dieter's Guide to White Wine

As you know by now, the great thing about the White Wine Diet is that you are allowed to drink two glasses of white wine every day, and eat some great food too. So why not make the most of it and enjoy the anticipation of these daily treats by choosing your wine carefully and really using the period you are on the diet to learn something about the great choice of white wine there is out there.

What follows is a brief rundown of the major white wine grape varieties to help you choose what will perfectly complement the meal choices you make. You'll see in the recipe section that I've made a wine selection for each recipe, but that's not set in stone. Pick and choose – experiment. It'll make the dieting a lot more fun!

Grape Varieties

This list is by no means exhaustive, but it covers most of the grape varieties the casual drinker is likely to encounter.

Chardonnay

Chardonnay is perhaps the most famous grape of all; certainly it is the most common, and many people adore it for its fruity taste, rich with apple, melon, pineapple and citrus flavours. It's a versatile grape, too, which when aged in oak produces more sophisticated tastes of vanilla and spices. A mainstay of the white wines of Burgundy – glass of Chablis, anyone? – it is also a common and important component of champagne.

Sauvignon Blanc

Sancerre and Pouilly-Fumé are the tipples of superstars, and both are made from the sophisticated Sauvignon Blanc grape. For the rest of us who want to enjoy the richly flavoured taste of this fantastic grape, the wines of New Zealand are a good place to start. It's also used in Bordeaux and, along with Semillon, is used to make Sauternes, the fabulous – if expensive – dessert wine. Look out for tropical fruits and gooseberries.

Riesling

Most famously grown in Germany, Riesling is used to produce some of the best wines in the world – although you do need to avoid some mass-produced 'brand' wines, which claim to be Riesling and are, in fact, rather unpleasant and over-sweet. It's also grown in Alsace and Australia, and is redolent with the fruity aroma and taste of limes, blossom and apples.

Semillon
Semillon is not widely grown. You'll find it in Bordeaux (as we've learned above, it is used in the making of Sauternes) and latterly in parts of Australia. It is prized for its honeyed, buttery taste, which becomes more complex as it is left to mature.

Chenin Blanc
Chenin Blanc comes into its own in the production of sweet wines, where it produces tastes of quince and honey, although you will find some dry whites made with this grape. Mostly cultivated in the Loire Valley, it is also to be found in South Africa, where it is called Steen.

Pinot Gris
Mostly grown in Alsace, Pinot Gris produces a spicy, flavoursome wine. In Italy it's known as Pinot Grigio, and is well prized.

Gewurztraminer
Another stalwart of the Alsace region, Gewurztraminer can be an acquired taste. Its champions wax lyrical about the banana and spice to be found in its complex taste.

Muscat

Mostly harvested for the production of the famous sweet wine, Muscat gives an orangey, citrusy hit along with the essential mustiness of a good sweet wine.

5
The White Wine
Diet Recipes

This is the fun bit! I've designed these recipes for people who love good food that will go well with a glass of wine, but don't want to spend hours and hours preparing it.

I hope there is something for everyone in the meals that follow: whether you need something to take to work (Lunch Box Humous and Crudités page 107), a quick-fix snack (BLT Treat, page 89) or something a little more elaborate for a dinner party or special occasion (Monkfish with a Trio of Vegetables, page 97), I've no doubt that you will find plenty here to tickle your tastebuds while slimming down.

And don't forget that the beauty of the White Wine Diet is that you are allowed two glasses a day of your favourite white wine (or even red wine, if you prefer). Whoever said dieting couldn't be enjoyable?

These recipes are divided into three sections: breakfasts, main meals (suitable for lunch or dinner) and desserts. It doesn't really matter what you eat when – although I would say that a sensible dieting tactic is to eat lighter meals at night – just so long as you are eating the correct number of calories. And don't be tempted to cut out breakfast so that you can eat more food later in the day. Breakfast is really important, and, if you skip it, you'll only be plagued by the mid-morning munchies …

Breakfasts

Black tea or coffee, sweetened if necessary with sweetener, may be included each morning.

25g low-fat, unsweetened cereal such as Shreddies served with 150ml skimmed milk
30g wholegrain bread toasted and topped with one small organic banana
(260 calories)

120g strawberries served with 150ml low-fat yogurt
1 wholewheat buttermilk pancake served with 1 teaspoon honey
(180 calories)

200ml fresh orange juice
1 poached egg on 30g wholegrain bread toasted and spread with ½ teaspoon of low-fat spread
1 apple (120g)
(291 calories)

60g tinned prunes
30g wholegrain bread toasted and topped with 60g cottage cheese and 1 medium sliced tomato
(195 calories)

The White Wine Diet

30g unsweetened muesli served with 150ml
skimmed milk
30g very lean boiled ham served with 60g grilled
fresh pineapple
(240 calories)

120g fresh grapefruit
45g (drained weight) sardines in brine spread on
30g wholegrain toast
(172 calories)

60g pork sausage (usually 1 sausage) grilled and surface
fat removed with kitchen paper. Serve with 100g low-
fat baked beans
1 medium orange
(295 calories)

Main Meals

RECIPES UNDER 100 CALORIES

Herb and Watercress Soup

Serves 4
60 calories per serving
Wine suggestion: Chardonnay

2 teaspoons margarine
1 bunch spring onions, trimmed and finely chopped
900ml vegetable stock
1 bunch watercress, trimmed and chopped
3 tablespoons fresh mixed herbs, chopped
1 tablespoon cornflour
2 tablespoons skimmed milk
salt and freshly ground black pepper

Melt the margarine in a large pan and cook the spring onions for 5 minutes over a medium heat, stirring occasionally until softened but not brown. Add the vegetable stock, watercress and herbs. Bring to the boil, reduce the heat and simmer, covered, for 10–15 minutes.

Transfer the soup to a liquidiser and blend for about 20 seconds until smooth. Return to the pan and reheat gently.

Blend the cornflour with the milk, add to the soup and heat gently, stirring constantly, until smooth and thickened. Taste and season with salt and pepper, if needed, and garnish with a few herbs before serving.

Oriental Chicken Soup

Serves 4
70 calories per serving
Wine suggestion: Pinot Gris

2 chicken stock cubes
900ml boiling water
1 leek, shredded
1 carrot, cut into sticks
1 bunch spring onions, finely sliced
½ teaspoon Chinese five-spice powder
1 teaspoon root ginger, grated
2 tablespoons light soy sauce
60g cooked lean chicken, shredded into fine strips
5cm piece cucumber, cut into fine strips
1 tablespoon fresh coriander, chopped
salt and freshly ground black pepper
1 teaspoon sesame seeds, lightly toasted

Dissolve the stock cubes in the water. Add the leek, carrot, spring onions, five-spice powder and ginger. Cover and simmer gently for 15 minutes. Add the soy sauce, shredded chicken, cucumber and coriander to the pan and simmer gently for a further 5 minutes. Season to taste. Ladle the soup into warmed bowls and sprinkle with the toasted sesame seeds.

Salmon Pâté

Serves 6
75 calories per serving
Wine suggestion: Gewurztraminer

1 tablespoon powdered gelatine
90ml very hot water
160g canned salmon
10cm piece cucumber, finely chopped
150ml vegetable stock
150ml low-fat natural yogurt
1 tablespoon fresh dill or parsley, chopped
6 x 30g slices wholemeal bread, toasted and cut
   into triangles
salt and freshly ground black pepper
herbs to garnish

Sprinkle the gelatine over the very hot (not boiling) water.
Stir well to dissolve. Ensure that the liquid is clear and
allow to cool for 10 minutes.

Mash the salmon in a bowl. Add the cucumber,
vegetable stock, yogurt and the herbs. Season with salt
and pepper. Transfer the mixture to a 900ml mould and
refrigerate until set (about 1½ hours).

To turn out the pâté, carefully ease a knife around the
edge. Dip the mould into warm water for a few seconds.
Place an inverted plate on top of the mould and flip over.
Shake gently to release the pâté. Slice the pâté and garnish.
Serve with the triangles of wholemeal toast.

Leek and Butterbean Broth

Serves 4
95 calories per serving
Wine suggestion: Chardonnay

2 teaspoons vegetable oil
2 large leeks, trimmed and chopped
1 large onion, finely chopped
900ml vegetable stock
1½ teaspoons Marmite
180g tinned butterbeans
2 tablespoons parsley, chopped
salt and freshly ground black pepper

Heat the oil in a large pan and sauté the leeks and onion for 3–4 minutes until softened. Add the stock and Marmite, stirring until dissolved. Bring to the boil, reduce and simmer, covered, for 20 minutes

Add the butterbeans and half the parsley, and cook gently for a further 5 minutes to warm through. Season to taste. The soup may be served as it is or liquidised for a smoother effect.

RECIPES UNDER 200 CALORIES

Baked Stuffed Mushrooms

Serves 4
135 calories per serving
Wine suggestion: Sauvignon Blanc

4 large flat mushrooms
2 garlic cloves
rind of 1 lemon, finely grated
40g wholemeal breadcrumbs
1 tablespoon parsley, chopped
1 tablespoon any other herbs, chopped
3 tablespoons virgin olive oil
salt and freshly ground black pepper
fresh parsley and lemon wedges to garnish

Wipe the mushrooms with a damp cloth. Carefully remove the stalks and chop them finely. Crush the garlic and place in a bowl with the lemon rind and the mushrooms, breadcrumbs, herbs and 1½ tablespoons of the oil. Add salt and freshly ground black pepper to taste, then stir well to mix all the ingredients.

Brush the bottom of a shallow ovenproof dish with 2 teaspoons of oil. Arrange the mushrooms in a single layer in the dish. Divide the stuffing equally among the mushrooms and sprinkle over the remaining oil. Bake in the oven for 15 minutes. Serve hot, garnished with the parsley and lemon.

Chicken Surprise Roll-Ups

Serves 4
135 calories per serving
Wine suggestion: Gewurztraminer

2 tablespoons low-fat natural yogurt
1 teaspoon mild curry powder
60g cooked chicken, chopped
½ medium banana
squeeze of lemon juice
4 slices white or brown bread
4 teaspoons fruit chutney
2 teaspoons low-fat spread
salt and freshly ground black pepper
2 teaspoons toasted sesame seeds

In a medium-sized bowl, mix together the yogurt and curry powder. Add the chicken, banana and lemon juice, stirring well to combine. Season to taste.

Spread each slice of bread with 1 teaspoon of chutney. Divide the chicken mixture equally between the slices and spread out evenly. Roll up neatly into sausage shapes. Spread ½ teaspoon of low-fat spread along the top of each and sprinkle with toasted sesame seeds.

Three-Bean Salad with Citrus Dressing

Serves 4
145 calories per serving
Wine suggestion: Chardonnay

240g dwarf green beans, trimmed and sliced
2 shallots, finely chopped
3 medium tomatoes, chopped
180g tinned red kidney beans, rinsed and drained
180g tinned soya beans, rinsed and drained

For the dressing
finely grated rind and juice of 1 small lemon
1 tablespoon white wine vinegar
2 tablespoons tomato purée
½ teaspoon paprika
1 tablespoon mint, chopped
salt and freshly ground black pepper
sprigs of fresh mint to garnish

Cook the green beans in a small amount of lightly salted water for 8–10 minutes until just tender. Drain and refresh under cold running water. Then make the dressing by mixing together the lemon rind and juice, vinegar, tomato purée, paprika, mint and seasoning.

Mix together the onion, tomatoes, kidney beans, soya beans and cooked green beans. Pour over the dressing and stir gently until combined. Divide the salad between 4 plates. Garnish with the fresh mint leaves.

Ottoman Salad

Serves 4
150 calories per serving
Wine suggestion: Sauvignon Blanc

115g crisp lettuce
50g rocket leaves
3 medium tomatoes
115g cucumber
25g spring onions
115g feta cheese
8 small sprigs mint

For the dressing
2 tablespoons olive oil
2 teaspoons lemon juice
1 teaspoon brown sugar
pinch of mustard powder
salt and freshly ground black pepper

Wash the salad leaves and pat dry, then tear them into bite-size pieces. Wash all the remaining salad vegetables. Slice the tomatoes, cucumber and onion into slices and dice. Arrange the salad leaves in a bowl and sprinkle the chopped ingredients on top. Stone and slice the olives and crumble the feta cheese. Chop half the mint and sprinkle it over the salad along with the olives and feta. Combine the salad dressing ingredients and pour over the salad. Garnish with the remaining mint sprigs.

Creamed Mushrooms on Wholemeal Toast

Serves 4
155 calories per serving
Wine suggestion: Semillon

360g button mushrooms
300ml skimmed milk
1 tablespoon fresh parsley, chopped
2 tablespoons cornflour
120g low-fat fromage frais
4 x 30g slices of wholemeal bread
salt and freshly ground black pepper
parsley to garnish

Put the mushrooms in a pan. Reserve 4 tablespoons of milk and add the rest to the pan together with the parsley. Simmer gently for 10 minutes.

Mix the cornflour with the reserved milk until smooth and blended. Add to the mushroom mixture and heat gently, stirring constantly until thickened. Simmer gently for 1 minute.

Spoon the fromage frais into the pan and fold into the mushrooms. Cook for 2 minutes to heat through, stirring occasionally. Season to taste.

Toast the bread and spoon the mushroom sauce on top. Serve at once garnished with the parsley.

German Sausage and Vegetable Chowder

Serves 4
160 calories per serving
Wine suggestion: Riesling

4 teaspoons margarine
1 large onion, finely chopped
1 large carrot, finely sliced
180g turnip, diced
900ml vegetable stock
120g frankfurters, sliced
½ teaspoon caraway seeds
1 tablespoon parsley, chopped
90g white or spring cabbage, finely shredded
salt and freshly ground black pepper

Melt the margarine in a large saucepan and sauté the vegetables for 3–4 minutes. Add the stock and bring to the boil. Reduce the heat and simmer, covered, for 20 minutes.

Add the frankfurters, caraway seeds, parsley and cabbage to the saucepan. Cover and cook gently for 10 more minutes. Season the chowder to taste and serve.

Garden Vegetable Soup

Serves 6
165 calories per serving
Wine suggestion: Chardonnay

4 medium carrots, cut into small chunks
4 medium leeks, trimmed and thinly sliced
4 small parsnips, cut into small chunks
4 celery sticks, strings removed with a potato peeler
   and thinly sliced
1 large onion, thinly sliced
1 swede, cut into small chunks
240g green cabbage, finely sliced
2 x 400g cans chopped tomatoes
3 large garlic cloves, crushed
2 bay leaves
3 teaspoons salt
4 litres vegetable stock
100g small pasta shells
2 level teaspoons dried mixed herbs
freshly ground black pepper

Place all the vegetables and the tomatoes in a large stock pan. Add the bay leaf, the salt and the stock. Bring to the boil and simmer for 25 minutes until tender. Add the pasta and the dried mixed herbs and cook for a further 15–20 minutes.

Remove the bay leaves and season to taste. The soup can be either wholly or partially liquidised. Serve very hot.

Thai Prawn Salad

Serves 4
165 calories per serving
Wine suggestion: Pinot Gris

250g packet cooked tiger prawns in their shells
140g bean sprouts
1 bunch radishes, thinly sliced
4 sticks celery, sliced
1 bunch spring onions, thinly sliced on the slant
300g combination of sugar snap peas,
   baby carrots and baby corn
1 lettuce
25g roasted salted peanuts, chopped

For the dressing
2 limes
2 tablespoons sunflower oil
2 teaspoons fish sauce
1 garlic clove, finely chopped
4 teaspoons sugar

To make the dressing, finely grate the zest of 1 lime and squeeze the juice from both limes. Mix the zest and juice together with the remaining dressing ingredients.

Peel the prawns, leaving the tails on, then tip them into a bowl and pour in one-third of the dressing. Put aside to allow the flavours to develop.

Toss together the bean sprouts, radishes, celery and

38

spring onions. Halve the sugar snap peas lengthways, thinly slice the carrots and corn and toss with the bean sprout mixture. Gently toss in the prawns and the remaining dressing.

Lay a bed of lettuce on a large platter and spoon the salad on top. Serve sprinkled with the peanuts.

Mushroom Omelette

Serves 2
165 calories per serving
Wine suggestion: Chardonnay

225g mushrooms, sliced
2 shallots, finely chopped
3 large eggs
3 tablespoons skimmed milk
2 teaspoons Mushroom ketchup (optional)
freshly ground black pepper

Dry-fry the mushrooms and shallots in a hot non-stick pan for 2–3 minutes until slightly coloured. Season well with the pepper.

Whisk the eggs together with the milk and ketchup. Pour on to the mushroom mixture, reduce the heat and cook until the omelette is just set. Fold in half and divide between 2 warm plates.

Lamb and Barley Broth

Serves 4
170 calories per serving
Wine suggestion: Riesling

240g best end neck of lamb, trimmed of fat
1 large onion, chopped
1 large carrot, chopped
1 leek, trimmed and finely sliced
180g swede, chopped
45g pearl barley
2 bay leaves
2 lamb stock cubes
1.2 litres boiling water
60g frozen peas
salt and freshly ground black pepper
1 tablespoon parsley, chopped

Place the pieces of lamb on the rack of a grill pan and grill until the fat stops dripping, turning once during cooking. Transfer to a large pan and add the onion, carrot, leek, swede, pearl barley and bay leaves. Dissolve the stock cubes in the boiling water and add to the pan. Bring to the boil and then reduce the heat. Cover and simmer gently for about 1 ½ hours until the meat is very tender.

Lift the lamb pieces from the broth, trim off the meat and discard the bones. Return the lamb to the pan. Add the frozen peas and reheat gently. Cook for about 3 minutes.

Season and serve, sprinkled with parsley.

Egg, Cucumber and Cannellini Salad with Paprika Dressing

Serves 4
195 calories per serving
Wine suggestion: Pinot Gris

1 bunch spring onions, finely chopped
4 sticks celery, finely sliced
10cm piece cucumber, chopped
360g tinned cannellini beans, rinsed and drained
4 hard-boiled eggs, quartered
1 tablespoon fresh parsley, chopped
150ml low-fat natural yogurt
1 tablespoon lemon juice
1 teaspoon ground paprika
salt and freshly ground black pepper
herbs to garnish

Mix together the spring onions, celery, cucumber and cannellini beans. Season with salt and pepper. Divide between 4 plates and arrange the hard-boiled eggs on top. Sprinkle with the chopped parsley.

Mix together the yogurt, lemon juice and most of the paprika in a small jug. Season with a little salt, then drizzle over the salads. Sprinkle with the rest of the paprika and garnish with the herbs.

You may substitute any variety of tinned beans (drained) in place of the cannellini beans.

RECIPES UNDER 300 CALORIES

Asian Vegetable Stir-Fry with Tofu

Serves 4
200 calories per serving
Wine suggestion: Pinot Gris

4 teaspoons sesame oil
30g unsalted peanuts
2 garlic cloves, crushed
1 small green chilli, finely chopped
4 shallots, peeled and sliced
1 yellow pepper, seeded and cut into strips
1 large carrot, cut into matchsticks
180g broccoli, broken into small florets
180g mushrooms, wiped and sliced
180g Chinese leaves, shredded
1 teaspoon ground ginger
1 teaspoon ground coriander
300g smoked or firm tofu, cut into cubes
salt and freshly ground black pepper

Heat the oil in a wok and add the peanuts. Stir-fry for about 1 minute until browned. Lift out and drain on kitchen paper. Set aside. Add the garlic and chilli to the wok and stir-fry for a few seconds. Now add all the remaining vegetables except the Chinese leaves. Stir-fry for about 3 minutes and then add the Chinese leaves, ginger, coriander and tofu. Stir-fry for 2 more minutes.

Season, sprinkle with the nuts and serve at once.

Warm Duck Salad

Serves 6
205 calories per serving
Wine suggestion: Pinot Gris

2 duck breasts
12 medium mushrooms
2 tablespoons extra virgin olive oil
15g unsalted butter
1 garlic clove
½ teaspoon balsamic vinegar
1 tablespoon lemon juice
1 small radicchio lettuce
1 bunch watercress
1 head of curly endive or escarole
1 tablespoon parsley, chopped
1 tablespoons basil, torn into pieces

For the marinade
2 shallots, finely chopped
1 tablespoon lemon juice
1 tablespoon extra virgin olive oil
1 tablespoon mixed herbs, chopped

Skin the duck and cut into long, thin slices. Mix all the marinade ingredients together in a large bowl, seasoning generously. Place the duck strips into the marinade and refrigerate for at least 1 hour (preferably overnight).

Wipe the mushrooms clean and slice them thinly.

44

Drain the duck strips and reserve the marinade. Heat the oil and the butter in a pan, add the duck strips and sauté for 2–3 minutes. Quickly transfer the duck to a separate dish and add the mushrooms to the pan. Sauté for 2–3 minutes over a high heat, stirring occasionally.

Peel and slice the garlic. Add the marinade to the mushrooms with the garlic, vinegar and lemon juice. Reduce the mixture by boiling for 2 minutes. Return the duck to the pan, coating the strips with the mixture. Remove from the heat.

Wash and dry the salad leaves, divide them between six plates and top with the duck strips. Pour the dressing over the salads. Garnish with parsley.

French Lunch

Serves 4
210 calories per serving
Wine suggestion: Chardonnay

1.2 litres live mussels
1 tablespoon margarine
2 garlic cloves, crushed
2 shallots, very finely chopped
2 tablespoons fresh parsley, chopped
finely grated rind and juice of 1 lemon
240ml hot vegetable stock
90ml dry white wine
salt and freshly ground black pepper
fresh parsley, chopped, and lemon slices to garnish
4 x 30g slices French bread to serve

Using a small, sharp knife, scrape the 'beards' off the mussels under cold running water. Scrub them well and discard any that are damaged or remain open when tapped. Keep rinsing until there is no trace of sand.

Melt the margarine in a large saucepan and sauté the garlic and shallots until softened but not coloured. Add the parsley, lemon rind and juice, hot vegetable stock and mussels. Put the lid on the pan and cook over a moderate heat so that the mussels steam for 3–5 minutes. Shake the pan from time to time.

Check that all the mussels have opened and discard any that remain shut. Lift out on to 4 warmed soup plates with a slotted spoon. Boil the remaining liquid rapidly together with the wine so that it reduces slightly, and then pour over the mussels. Season, garnish with parsley and lemon slices, and serve with the French bread to mop up the juices.

Pan-Fried Summer Vegetables with Eggs

Serves 4
215 calories per serving
Wine suggestion: Semillon

2 tablespoons olive oil
1 onion, finely chopped
1 red chilli, seeded and finely chopped
2 large red peppers, seeded and sliced
2 large yellow peppers, seeded and sliced
2 large courgettes, diced
3 plum tomatoes, diced
1 teaspoon mixed herbs
4 medium fresh eggs
salt and freshly ground black pepper

Heat the oil in a large frying pan and add the onion, chilli, peppers and courgettes. Cook, stirring frequently, until softened.

Add the tomatoes, herbs and seasoning and continue to cook for a further 5 minutes.

Make 4 hollows in the mixture with the back of a spoon and carefully break an egg into each one. Continue cooking over a low heat until the eggs are just set.

Welsh Potato Cakes

Serves 4
215 calories per serving
Wine suggestion: Gewurztraminer

1 large leek, trimmed and finely chopped
1 small onion, finely chopped
90g Caerphilly cheese, grated
480g cooled mashed potato
1 tablespoon chives or parsley, chopped
1 beaten egg
2 tablespoons water
60g fresh breadcrumbs
salt and freshly ground black pepper

Preheat the oven to 190°C/Gas 5. Cook the leek and onion in a small amount of lightly salted boiling water for about 10 minutes or until tender. Drain well.

In a large mixing bowl, combine the leeks and onion with the cheese, mashed potato and chives or parsley. Season to taste with salt and pepper. Form the mixture into 8 evenly sized cakes.

Beat the egg and water together on a shallow plate. Put the breadcrumbs on another plate. Brush each potato cake with the egg mixture and then coat with the breadcrumbs. Place on a non-stick baking sheet.

Bake in the oven for 15–20 minutes until light golden-brown and crisp on the outside.

Pasta Shapes with Tomato Sauce

Serves 4
215 calories per serving
Wine suggestion: Chenin Blanc

2 teaspoons olive oil
1 medium onion, finely chopped
420g very ripe tomatoes, skinned and chopped
   (or use tinned tomatoes)
1 tablespoon basil or oregano, chopped
   (or use 1 teaspoon dried)
4–5 tablespoons water
180g pasta shapes
4 teaspoons grated Parmesan cheese
salt and freshly ground black pepper
sprigs of fresh basil to garnish

Heat the oil in a pan and sauté the onion for 4–5 minutes until softened. Add the tomatoes, basil or oregano and water, stirring well. Cover and cook over a low heat for 15–20 minutes, stirring from time to time. Add a little extra water if required – the sauce should be thick and pulpy.

Cook the pasta in plenty of lightly salted boiling water until *al dente*. Drain well, then add to the sauce, stirring to coat. Season with salt and pepper. Divide the pasta and sauce between 4 warmed plates. Sprinkle 1 teaspoon of Parmesan cheese on top of each one and garnish with fresh herbs.

Chicken and Vegetable Curry with Lentils

Serves 4
215 calories per serving
Wine suggestion: Pinot Gris

1 tablespoon vegetable oil
2 garlic cloves
1 large onion, sliced
2 sticks celery, sliced
1 large carrot, sliced
1 medium courgette, sliced
2 tablespoons medium curry powder, or mild if preferred
900ml freshly made vegetable stock (or use stock cubes)
1 tablespoon tomato purée
120g red lentils
4 x 120g skinned chicken thighs
2 tablespoons mint, chopped
150ml low-fat natural yogurt
salt and freshly ground black pepper
fresh herbs to garnish

Heat the oil in a large pan and sauté the garlic and onion for 3 minutes. Add the celery, carrot and courgette, and cook for a further 2 minutes.

Sprinkle the curry powder into the saucepan and stir well to coat the vegetables. Cook gently for 1 minute.

Cover the vegetables with the stock and add the tomato purée. Bring to the boil and reduce the heat. Add the lentils and chicken and cover the pan. Simmer over a low heat for about 45 minutes, stirring from time to time. Taste the curry and season with salt and pepper.

Mix the mint into the yogurt and serve as an accompaniment to the curry. Garnish with mint sprigs.

Fishy Soufflé Omelettes

Serves 4
215 calories per serving
Wine suggestion: Sauvignon Blanc

120g tinned crab, drained and flaked
120g low-fat fromage frais
1 tablespoon tomato purée
6 eggs, separated
2 tablespoons watercress leaves, finely chopped
4 teaspoons vegetable oil
salt and freshly ground black pepper
watercress sprigs to garnish

Combine the crabmeat, fromage frais and tomato purée in a small saucepan over a very low heat, stirring gently. Season with salt and pepper then set aside. Beat the egg yolks in a large mixing bowl and add the chopped watercress. Season and stir. In a large grease-free bowl, whisk the egg whites until they hold their shape and fold them gently into the egg yolk mixture, using a large metal spoon.

Heat the grill. Cooking one omelette at a time, heat 1 teaspoon of oil in a small omelette pan. Add one quarter of the egg mixture and cook on the stove for 1–2 minutes until the base is set. Place under the grill for a few seconds to set the top.

Put on a warmed plate and spoon on a quarter of the crab mixture. Fold and serve, garnished with the watercress.

American Combination Salad

Serves 4
215 calories per serving
Wine suggestion: Chardonnay

50g whole fresh almonds, shelled
225g young spinach
450g ripe strawberries
1 bulb fennel

For the dressing
juice of ½ orange
1 teaspoon Dijon mustard
2 tablespoons virgin olive oil
1 tablespoon white balsamic or white wine vinegar
salt and freshly ground black pepper

Preheat the oven to 200°C/Gas 6. Roast the almonds on a baking tray in the oven for about 7 minutes, checking frequently to avoid burning. Tip into a bowl.

Wash the spinach and pat dry. Discard any coarse leaves or stems. Wash, hull and halve the strawberries. Remove the feathery tops and hard base from the fennel and cut into very thin strips.

Put all the dressing ingredients into a screw-top jar and shake well. Taste and adjust the seasoning. Combine the salad ingredients in a large bowl, pour over the dressing and toss gently.

Chicken Drumsticks with Lemon and Ginger Coating

Serves 4
220 calories per serving
Wine suggestion: Chardonnay

8 x 75g skinned chicken drumsticks
60g wholemeal flour
rind of 1 small lemon, finely grated
¼ teaspoon ground ginger
¼ teaspoon ground cumin
salt and freshly ground black pepper
lemon slices to garnish

Preheat the oven to 190°C/Gas 5. Rinse the drumsticks, but do not pat dry. Put the flour, lemon rind, ginger, cumin and seasoning into a large polythene bag and shake well to mix. Put the drumsticks into the bag, seal and shake so that they are well coated in the seasoned flour.

Arrange the drumsticks on a non-stick baking sheet and cook in the oven for 20–25 minutes. Check that they are cooked by piercing with a skewer in the thickest part, making sure that the juices run clear. Garnish with the lemon slices and serve with a mixed salad.

Salmon Fishcakes

Serves 4
220 calories per portion
Wine suggestion: Chardonnay

210g tinned red salmon
2 spring onions, roughly chopped
360g cooked mashed potato
2 tablespoons fresh parsley, chopped
30g wholemeal plain flour
1 egg, beaten
2 tablespoons water
45g dried breadcrumbs
salt and freshly ground black pepper

Preheat the oven to 190°C/Gas 5. Put the salmon, spring onions, cooked potato, parsley and seasoning into a food processor and blend for a few seconds until combined but not too smooth. Form the mixture into 8 small fishcakes.

Lightly coat each cake with the flour and then dip each one into the egg and water mixture, and finally coat with the breadcrumbs. Place on a non-stick baking sheet and bake for 20 minutes until hot and crisp on the outside.

Meat and Vegetable Steamed Puddings

Serves 4
225 calories per serving
Wine suggestion: Pinot Gris

½ teaspoon vegetable oil
240g lean minced beef
1 small onion, finely chopped
1 small carrot, grated
1 small turnip, grated
60g fresh white breadcrumbs
1 tablespoon mixed herbs, chopped, or 1
  teaspoon dried
salt and freshly ground black pepper
1 egg, beaten

For the gravy
1½ teaspoons margarine
1 medium onion, chopped
300ml hot water
1 beef stock cube
2 teaspoons cornflour blended with a little water

Brush 4 individual pudding basins with the vegetable oil. Form the minced beef into small patties and place them on a grill rack. Grill them, turning once, until the fat stops dripping. Cool and then crumble.

In a large mixing bowl, combine the onion, carrot, turnip, minced beef, breadcrumbs, herbs and seasoning.

Add the egg and mix thoroughly. Divide between the basins, cover with foil and steam for 1 hour.

Melt the margarine in a saucepan and sauté the onion until well browned. Add the hot water and stock cube, stirring to dissolve. Simmer for 10 minutes and then add the blended cornflour, stirring until thickened. Cook for 1 minute. Check the seasoning.

Turn out the puddings and pour over a little of the gravy.

Smoked Chicken Salad

Serves 4
230 calories per serving
Wine suggestion: Pinot Gris

2 smoked chicken breasts, skinned and boneless
1 tablespoon virgin olive oil
350g fresh young spinach
175g button mushrooms
4 spring onions
1 large ripe avocado
squeeze of lemon

For the dressing
1 garlic clove
4 tablespoons natural yogurt
juice of 1 orange
1½ teaspoons white wine vinegar
1 teaspoon Dijon mustard
½ teaspoon Tabasco sauce
2 tablespoons parsley, chopped

Preheat the oven to 190°C/Gas 5. Put the chicken breasts on an oiled baking tray and cook for 10 minutes on each side. Meanwhile, wash and dry the spinach.

To make the dressing, chop or crush the garlic and mix all the ingredients, apart from the parsley, and season with plenty of black pepper.

Prepare and slice the mushrooms. Trim and slice the

spring onions. Cut the avocado in half, dice the flesh into 20mm cubes and sprinkle with the lemon juice to stop the avocado discolouring.

When the chicken is cooked, cut it into bite-size chunks and stir any juices into the dressing. While the chicken is still warm, mix all the ingredients for the salad in a large bowl. Sprinkle with the parsley and serve the dressing separately in a small jug.

Avocado and Citrus Salad

Serves 4
230 calories per serving
Wine suggestion: Chardonnay

3 large oranges
½ cucumber
1 large avocado
fresh herbs to garnish

For the dressing
3 tablespoons fresh orange juice
1 tablespoon red wine vinegar
1 teaspoon grain mustard
1 tablespoon virgin olive oil
2 teaspoons snipped chives
salt and freshly ground black pepper

Remove the peel and the pith from the oranges and, cutting between the membranes, remove the segments neatly. Wipe the cucumber and cut in half lengthways. Remove the seeds and slice the cucumber thinly into neat crescent shapes. Cut the avocado in half and remove the stone. Peel and dice the flesh. Place the dressing ingredients into a bowl and whisk together well. Add the avocado and mix gently to coat it in the dressing.

Serve on 4 plates, alternating slices of orange and cucumber with the avocado in the middle. Spoon over the dressing. Garnish with the herbs.

Hungarian Goulash

Serves 4
230 calories per serving
Wine suggestion: Pinot Gris

360g lean stewing steak, in one piece
2 teaspoons vegetable oil
1 large onion, sliced
1 large garlic clove, crushed
1 tablespoon paprika
420g tinned tomatoes, chopped
1 tablespoon tomato purée
1 large red pepper, seeded and chopped
1 beef stock cube dissolved in 600ml hot water
1 tablespoon cornflour, blended with a little water
4 tablespoons low-fat natural yogurt
salt and freshly ground black pepper
fresh parsley, chopped, to garnish

Put the piece of steak on a grill rack and grill until the fat stops dripping, turning once. Cool and then cut into 2.5cm cubes.

Heat the oil in a large pan and sauté the onion and garlic for 3–5 minutes until softened. Add the paprika, stirring well.

Add the tomatoes, tomato purée, red pepper, meat and stock to the pan. Bring to the boil and reduce the heat. Cover and simmer for 1–1½ hours until the meat is tender. Check the level of liquid from time to time, topping up with a little extra water or stock if necessary.

Season the goulash with salt and pepper. Add the blended cornflour and stir until thickened. Cook for 1 minute. Serve with 1 tablespoon of yogurt per portion and sprinkle with parsley. This would be good served with some rice, but remember to add the calorie content to your daily intake.

Crab with Marinated Sweet Peppers in Filo Cases

Serves 4
235 calories per serving
Wine suggestion: Chenin Blanc

225g fresh white prepared crabmeat (or use tinned crabmeat)
watercress to garnish

For the marinade
2 large red peppers
2 garlic cloves
2 tablespoons virgin olive oil
2 tablespoons lemon juice
½ teaspoon runny honey
salt and freshly ground black pepper

For the tartlet cases
3 x 355x190mm sheets filo pastry
25g butter

Preheat the oven to 190°C/Gas 5. Lay the peppers on a baking tray and bake for 30 minutes until they are blackened and blistered. When cool, peel away the skin and discard the seeds. Cut into thin slices.

Peel and crush the garlic. Whisk together all the ingredients for the marinade and stir in the peppers. Leave covered in the refrigerator for about 1 hour.

Spread melted butter finely over one sheet of filo

64

pastry. Lay over a second sheet and brush again, and finally lay a third sheet on top. Stamp out 8 circles from the layered pastry and use them to line 8 individual patty tins. Prick the bottom of each and bake for 6–8 minutes until golden. Allow to cool before filling.

Break up the crabmeat and mix it in with the peppers and marinade. Divide this mixture between the filo cases and garnish with the watercress. These may be served cold or slightly warmed through.

Vegetable Omelette Wedges

Serves 4
240 calories per serving
Wine suggestion: Chenin Blanc

2 tablespoons olive oil
360g potatoes, peeled and cut into small cubes
2 large onions, chopped
2 garlic cloves, crushed
1 small red pepper, seeded and chopped
4 eggs, beaten
4 tablespoons skimmed milk
salt and freshly ground black pepper

In a medium-sized frying pan, gently heat the olive oil. Add the potatoes, onions and garlic and sauté for about 15 minutes, stirring occasionally until the potatoes are cooked and golden brown. Add the red pepper and cook gently for about 5 more minutes. Season to taste.

Preheat the grill. Beat the eggs and milk together and pour into the pan. Cook gently to set the base – it should take about 5 minutes – and then brown the top under the grill.

Turn out the omelette on to a warm plate and cut into 4 wedges. Serve with a crisp green salad.

Mediterranean Toasties

Serves 1
245 calories per serving
Wine suggestion: Riesling

2 thin slices of French bread, cut on the slant
1 small onion, thinly sliced
½ red pepper, seeded and finely sliced
1 large garlic clove, crushed
1 small courgette, finely sliced
75g mushrooms, sliced
2 medium tomatoes, skinned and chopped
1 teaspoon tomato paste dissolved in 90ml hot water
½ teaspoon dried mixed herbs
salt and freshly ground black pepper

Toast the bread. In a non-stick pan dry-fry the onions until soft. Add the pepper, garlic, courgette and mushrooms and cook briskly over a high heat, turning them constantly.

Add the tomatoes and the tomato paste and water mixture together with the dried herbs and simmer until the liquid has reduced to a spreadable paste.

Spread the mixture on to the toast and place under a hot grill until brown. Serve hot.

Sirloin Steak with Mustard and Peppercorn Sauce

Serves 4
260 calories per serving
Wine suggestion: Gewurztraminer

4 x 175g sirloin steaks
2 shallots, finely chopped
2 garlic cloves, finely chopped
1 teaspoon green peppercorns, crushed
2 teaspoons coarse grain mustard
2 tablespoons brandy
225ml Greek yogurt
juice of ½ lemon
salt and freshly ground black pepper.

Trim the steaks of any fat. Heat a griddle or heavy frying pan until very hot and spray with a little oil. Fry the steaks in the hot pan for 2 minutes on each side. Reduce the heat and cook for up to 2–3 minutes more. Eight minutes will give a well-done steak; reduce the cooking time by half for a rare steak. Keep warm.

Add the shallots and garlic to the pan juices. Cook over a low heat, stirring until lightly coloured. Add the crushed peppercorns, mustard and brandy. Stir in the yogurt and lemon juice. Heat gently without boiling and pour over the steaks.

Cottage Cheese and Fruity Coleslaw Sandwiches

Serves 4
265 calories per serving
Wine suggestion: Semillon

90g firm white cabbage, finely shredded
1 small onion, grated or finely chopped
1 small carrot, grated
30g sultanas or raisins
30g dried apricots, chopped
4 tablespoons low-fat natural yogurt
1 teaspoon lemon juice
8 x 30g slices of brown bread
120g low-fat cottage cheese
salt and freshly ground black pepper

In a bowl, combine the cabbage, onion, carrot, sultanas or raisins and apricots. Add the yogurt, lemon juice and season with salt and pepper, stirring well.

Spread each slice of bread with the cheese and pile an equal quantity of the coleslaw on to 4 slices. Top with the remaining bread and cut the sandwiches into triangles. Serve soon after making to avoid sogginess.

Crispy Potato Skins with Savoury Dip

Serves 4
275 calories per serving
Wine suggestion: Chardonnay

4 x 240g baking potatoes, scrubbed
1 beaten egg
4 tablespoons skimmed milk
2 teaspoons flour
salt and freshly ground black pepper

For the dip
240g low-fat fromage frais
4 spring onions, finely chopped
1–2 garlic cloves, crushed
1 tablespoon fresh chives, chopped
pinch of celery salt

Preheat the oven to 200°C/Gas 6. Bake the potatoes for approximately 1 hour until cooked. Cool slightly, cut each one into quarters and scoop out some of the flesh, but leave a thickish layer close to the skin.

Beat the egg and milk together and brush all over the potato skins. Dust with the flour and place on a baking sheet. Season well. Return to the oven and bake for a further 15–20 minutes until crisp and golden brown.

Mix together the fromage frais, spring onions, garlic, chives and celery salt. Season with pepper and transfer to a small serving bowl. Serve as a dip with the hot potato skins.

Marinated Fish Fillets

Serves 4
280 calories per serving
Wine suggestion: Sauvignon Blanc

700g very fresh white fish fillets
1 medium onion
1 orange
4 limes
2 teaspoons oregano, chopped,
    or 1 teaspoon dried
2 tablespoons coriander, chopped
4 tablespoons virgin olive oil
1 teaspoon caster sugar
1 teaspoon Tabasco
1 large lettuce heart
salt and freshly ground black pepper
1 lime cut into wedges to serve

It is important that you choose the freshest fish you can find, as it is going to be cooked not using heat but using the citrus fruit.

Skin the fish and cut into bite-sized pieces. Chop the onion and place in a bowl with the fish. Squeeze the orange and 4 limes and pour the juice over the fish and onion. Cover and place in the refrigerator for at least 5 hours, until the fish is opaque.

Add the chopped herbs to the fish, along with the olive oil, caster sugar and Tabasco. Season to taste and mix thoroughly. Leave for 1 hour in a cool place, allowing the flavours to infuse.

Shred the lettuce and divide between 4 plates. Pile the marinated fish into the centre of the lettuce and serve with the lime wedges.

Crispy-Coated Liver and Onions

Serves 4
285 calories per serving
Wine suggestion: Gewurztraminer

1 medium onion, sliced into rings
60g wholemeal flour
30g cornflakes, finely crushed
450g lamb's liver, thinly sliced
150ml skimmed milk
salt and freshly ground black pepper

Put the onion rings in a bowl and pour over sufficient boiling water to cover. Leave for 5 minutes.

Mix together the flour and crushed cornflakes and sprinkle on to a plate. Season with salt and pepper. Dip the slices of liver into the milk, and then roll in the flour mixture. Place on a grill rack. Drain the onion rings, dust with the remaining flour mixture and arrange on the rack next to the liver.

Heat the grill and cook the liver and onions for 8–10 minutes, turning once until they are cooked and crisp.

Tomato Upside-Down Tart

Serves 4
295 calories per serving
Wine suggestion: Chardonnay

1 teaspoon olive oil
knob of butter
1 teaspoon caster sugar
about 10 tomatoes, halved widthways

For the pastry
100g plain flour
50g butter, chopped
50g mature Cheddar cheese, grated
4 spring onions, chopped

Preheat the oven to 180°C/Gas 4. Put the flour, butter and cheese in a food processor and blend to make crumbs. Add the spring onions and mix briefly. With the machine running, add 2–3 tablespoons of water and process until the mixture forms a ball. Wrap in cling film and set aside.

Heat a 23cm pan and add the oil and butter. Add the sugar and heat until caramelised, stirring it into the butter and oil. Pack the tomatoes into the pan, some skin side up and some skin side down. Cook over a high heat for a few minutes until the tomatoes start to colour on the underside. Remove from the heat and leave to cool.

Roll out the pastry until it is slightly larger than the pan. Put the pastry over the tomatoes and tuck the edges down the side of the pan. Bake for 15–20 minutes until the pastry is golden. Remove, cool for 5 minutes so the juices can settle, then invert on to a plate so the pastry is on the bottom. Cut into 4 and serve.

RECIPES UNDER 400 CALORIES

Noodles with Mushroom and Tomato Sauce

Serves 4
300 calories per serving
Wine suggestion: Sauvignon Blanc

2 teaspoons sesame or vegetable oil
1 large onion, chopped
1–2 garlic cloves, crushed
240g mushrooms, sliced
420g tinned tomatoes, chopped
150ml vegetable stock
2 tablespoons coriander or parsley, chopped
240g Chinese noodles
1 tablespoon soy sauce
1 tablespoon cornflour, blended with a little water
salt and freshly ground black pepper

Heat the oil in a medium-sized saucepan and sauté the onion and garlic together for 3–4 minutes until softened. Add the mushrooms, tomatoes, stock and coriander or parsley. Bring to the boil and then reduce the heat and simmer gently, uncovered, for 10–15 minutes to reduce slightly.

Pour boiling water over the Chinese noodles and allow to soak for approximately 6 minutes, or prepare according to pack instructions.

Add the soy sauce to the mushroom and tomato mixture, and season to taste with salt and pepper. Add the blended cornflour and cook for 2 minutes to thicken, stirring constantly.

Drain the noodles and divide between 4 warmed plates. Spoon the sauce on top and serve immediately.

Green Tagliatelle with Chicken and Artichoke Hearts

Serves 4
300 calories per serving
Wine suggestion: Semillon

2 tablespoons olive oil
1 large onion, finely chopped
2 tablespoons sherry vinegar
2 raw skinless chicken breasts, sliced into chunky strips
2 glasses dry white wine
juice of 1 lemon
1 tablespoon fresh tarragon, roughly chopped
400g tinned artichoke hearts, drained and cut into
    bite-sized pieces
4 tablespoons Greek yogurt
350g green tagliatelle
75g mangetout, trimmed and halved
115g broccoli florets
salt and freshly ground black pepper

Heat the oil in a pan and add the onion and the vinegar. Cook over a medium heat for about 3 minutes. Add the chicken and cook for another 3 minutes, stirring from time to time. Add the wine and the lemon juice and reduce the heat to a simmer.

Add the chopped tarragon leaves to the chicken together with the artichokes. Stir in the yogurt, adjust the seasoning and continue to simmer over a low heat.

Cook the pasta in a large pan according to the

instructions. Cook the mangetout and broccoli in boiling water until just tender. Drain the pasta and the vegetables. Spoon the chicken, artichokes and sauce on top of the pasta and arrange the vegetables around the dish.

Pasta with Chicken and Vegetables

Serves 4
300 calories per serving
Wine suggestion: Riesling

2 tablespoons extra virgin olive oil
2 tablespoons white wine vinegar (or white
 balsamic vinegar)
1 large onion, finely chopped
2 large uncooked skinless chicken breasts, cut into strips
2 glasses white wine
juice of 1 lemon
400g tinned artichoke hearts, drained and cut into
 bite-sized pieces
1 tablespoon fresh tarragon, chopped, or 1 teaspoon dried
4 tablespoon strained fat-free Greek yogurt
350g green tagliatelle
75g small mangetout
115g broccoli, broken into florets
salt and freshly ground black pepper

Heat the oil in a frying pan, add the vinegar and onion and
cook for 3 minutes over a medium heat. Add the chicken
and cook for a further 3 minutes, stirring occasionally.
Pour in the wine and the lemon juice and reduce the heat
so that the sauce is just simmering. Add the artichokes
and tarragon to the chicken. Stir in the yogurt, adjust the
seasoning and continue to simmer over a low heat.

Cook the pasta in a large pan of boiling salted water.

Cook the broccoli florets and mangetout in a smaller pan of boiling salted water for 2 or 3 minutes.

Drain the pasta and vegetables as soon as they are cooked. Spoon the chicken, artichokes and sauce over the pasta. Divide between 4 plates and arrange the green vegetables around the edge of the plates.

Braised Beef with Mushrooms

Serves 4
305 calories per serving
Wine suggestion: Chenin Blanc

700g braising steak, cut into 40mm cubes
2 large onions, quartered
115g button mushrooms
4 large carrots, cut crossways into 4
4 sticks celery, cut crossways into 4
½ teaspoon dried mixed herbs
1 bay leaf
1 tablespoon tomato purée
1 teaspoon brown sugar
570ml beef stock
285ml Guinness
1 tablespoon cornflour
1 tablespoon water
salt and freshly ground black pepper
chopped parsley

Preheat the oven to 160°C/Gas 3. Place the meat and vegetables in an ovenproof casserole along with the mixed herbs, bay leaf, tomato purée, sugar, beef stock and Guinness. Stir to mix thoroughly. Gently bring the stew to the boil, then cover and transfer to the oven. Cook very gently in the oven for about 2½ hours until the meat is quite tender.

Remove the meat. Mix the cornflour with 1 tablespoon

water until smooth, then stir into the casserole. Bring to the boil, stirring until thickened. Adjust seasoning to taste. Return the meat to the casserole and warm through gently. Transfer to a serving dish and sprinkle with the freshly chopped parsley.

Chinese-Style Beef and Vegetables

Serves 4
310 calories per serving
Wine suggestion: Riesling

8 x 50g slices entrecôte steak
50g leeks
50g carrots
50g green beans
50g young turnips
8 small shallots
4 tablespoons vegetable oil
1 tablespoon red wine vinegar
385ml red wine
150ml beef stock
1 tablespoon oyster sauce
1 tablespoon soy sauce
1½ teaspoons arrowroot or cornflour
1 tablespoon water

Trim all fat from the beef, and bat well with a rolling pin until quite thin. Cut all the vegetables, except the shallots, into thin strips. Plunge them into boiling water for 30 seconds to blanch and then drain.

Put the slices of beef on individual pieces of cling film and divide the vegetables over them. Now roll up each slice tightly in the cling film and screw up the overlapping film at the sides to tighten even further. When you unwrap the rolls they should have stuck together well.

Heat 1 tablespoon of the oil in a large frying pan over a medium heat and brown the beef rolls on all sides for about 5 minutes. Remove from the pan. Cut the shallots into thin rings. Add the remaining oil and the vinegar to the pan and sauté the shallots for about 5 minutes until they are transparent and the vinegar is reduced. Add the wine, stock, oyster sauce and soy sauce and bring to a simmer. Mix the arrowroot or cornflour with the water and stir into the sauce until thickened.

Return the beef rolls to the pan and simmer for 5 minutes. Remove to individual plates and cover with the sauce.

Salmon Tartare

Serves 4
310 calories per serving
Wine suggestion: Chardonnay

450g very fresh salmon
175g smoked salmon
2 tablespoons tarragon vinegar
salt and freshly ground black pepper
sprigs of dill

For the dill sauce
4 tablespoons reduced-calorie mayonnaise
4 tablespoons sour cream
2 tablespoons freshly chopped dill
1 tablespoon chopped chives
salt and freshly ground black pepper

Skin and bone the fresh salmon. Cut into small cubes and place in a bowl. Cut the smoked salmon into very fine strips and set aside. Add the vinegar to the bowl and season with a little salt, some dill and plenty of black pepper. Arrange the salmon on a serving platter with the fresh fish on one side and the smoked fish on the other.

To make the dill sauce, blend all the ingredients together in a bowl and serve separately.

Kidney and Vegetable Risotto

Serves 4
310 calories per serving
Wine suggestion: Pinot Gris

1 tablespoon olive oil
180g risotto or long-grain rice
1 medium onion, chopped
120g mushrooms, sliced
1 stick celery, sliced
1 small green pepper, seeded and chopped
30g plain flour
240g lamb's kidney, chopped
1 tablespoon fresh oregano, chopped,
  or 1 teaspoon dried
900ml vegetable stock
4 teaspoons grated Parmesan cheese
salt and freshly ground black pepper
parsley to garnish

Heat the oil in a large frying pan or wok. Add the rice and sauté for 5 minutes, then add the onion, mushrooms, celery and green pepper. Cook, stirring, for 5 minutes.

Sprinkle the flour on to a plate and season well with salt and pepper. Toss the kidney pieces in the flour, add to the frying pan with the oregano and stir through. Pour the stock into the pan and simmer the rice mixture over a low heat for 15–20 minutes until the rice is tender and the liquid has been absorbed. (If the liquid has been absorbed

before the rice is fully cooked, add a little extra water.)
Season to taste.

Divide the risotto between 4 warmed plates, sprinkle
with Parmesan cheese and garnish with parsley.

BLT Treat

Serves 1
310 calories per serving
Wine suggestion: Chardonnay

2 rashers of back bacon with all fat removed
1 iceberg lettuce
1 medium ripe plum tomato
2 baby gherkins
2 teaspoons low-fat mayonnaise
2 teaspoons tomato ketchup
¼ teaspoon Tabasco sauce
2 slices wholemeal bread

Grill the bacon on each side and place it on some kitchen paper to remove any fat. Shred the lettuce and slice the tomato and gherkins thinly. In a small bowl, mix together the mayonnaise, tomato ketchup and Tabasco sauce. Spread this mixture on both slices of bread. Layer the bread first with the lettuce and then the bacon followed by the tomatoes and gherkins. Cut in half and serve.

Plaice with Watercress Sauce

Serves 4
315 calories per serving
Wine suggestion: Chardonnay

1 small onion, finely chopped
15g butter
1 bunch watercress (or 1 large pack)
5 tablespoons single cream
25g soft low-fat cheese
8 small plaice fillets
2 tablespoons vegetable oil
salt and freshly ground black pepper
watercress sprigs to garnish
1 lemon

Gently sauté the onion in the butter for 5 minutes. Add the watercress and cook for a further 2 minutes until the watercress is wilted but retains its colour. Blend this mixture in a food processor and, while the motor is running, add the cream and the cheese. Blend until smooth.

Brush the plaice fillets lightly with oil and place on a lightly oiled baking tray. Season to taste and grill until lightly golden.

Gently reheat the sauce and divide between 4 plates. Dish the fish at the side and garnish with sprigs of watercress and a quarter of a lemon.

Cottage Cheese Combination Salad

Serves 4
315 calories per serving
Wine suggestion: Semillon

1 bunch watercress
4 medium oranges
480g cottage cheese
90g seedless grapes, halved
30g raisins
2 tablespoons sunflower seeds, toasted
2 tablespoons lemon juice
4 teaspoons olive or vegetable oil
salt and freshly ground black pepper

Wash the watercress and divide between 4 plates. Remove the zest from 2 of the oranges and put in a small jug. Remove the peel and pith from the oranges, using a sharp knife. Segment the oranges neatly and divide them between the plates on the other side of the watercress.

Mix together the cottage cheese, grapes, raisins and most of the sunflower seeds. Pile into the centre of the salads. Add the lemon juice and oil to the grated orange rind and mix well. Season with salt and pepper, and drizzle over the salads. Garnish with the reserved sunflower seeds.

Pasta and Vegetable Medley

Serves 4
320 calories per serving
Wine suggestion: Pinot Gris

180g broccoli, broken into small florets
1 large carrot, cut into matchsticks
1 onion, finely sliced
2 medium courgettes, finely sliced
120g mushrooms, sliced
240g pasta shapes
4 teaspoons margarine
1–2 garlic cloves, crushed
juice of 1 lemon
1 tablespoon tarragon or parsley, chopped
150ml vegetable stock
2 teaspoons cornflour, blended with a little water
4 teaspoons grated Parmesan cheese
salt and freshly ground black pepper
parsley to garnish

Steam the vegetables for about 10 minutes until tender.
Cook the pasta in plenty of lightly salted boiling water for
8–10 minutes until *al dente*.

Melt the margarine in a small pan, sauté the garlic for
2–3 minutes and then add the lemon juice, herbs and
stock. Heat until just boiling, and add the blended
cornflour, stirring until smooth and thickened. Cook for
1 minute and season to taste with salt and pepper.

Drain the pasta, add the vegetables and gently stir together. Season with a little salt and pepper. Serve on 4 warmed plates and drizzle the hot lemon and herb dressing equally over each portion. Sprinkle with the Parmesan cheese and garnish.

Kedgeree

Serves 4
320 calories per serving
Wine suggestion: Sauvignon Blanc

180g long-grain rice
480g smoked haddock fillet
2 teaspoons margarine
1 teaspoon cumin seeds
pinch of turmeric
1 large onion, finely chopped
2 eggs, hard boiled and chopped
2 tablespoons parsley, chopped
salt and freshly ground black pepper
parsley to garnish

Cook the rice in plenty of lightly salted boiling water for about 12 minutes until just tender. Rinse well in cold water and drain thoroughly.

Poach the fish in a large frying pan with just enough water to cover, until the flesh looks opaque and flakes easily. Drain well, discard any skin and bones, and flake the fish.

Melt the margarine in a large saucepan and gently sauté the cumin seeds, turmeric and onion for about 5 minutes. Add the rice and stir gently over a moderate heat for 3 minutes to heat through. Add the fish, chopped eggs and parsley. Season to taste with salt and pepper and cook for a further 2 minutes. Serve at once garnished with parsley.

Pineapple Salad with Bean Sprouts and Peanuts

Serves 4
330 calories per serving
Wine suggestion: Sauvignon Blanc

225g fresh or tinned pineapple in own juice
200g bean sprouts
2 medium carrots
½ large cucumber
4 spring onions
75g roasted peanuts

For the dressing
2 tablespoons crunchy peanut butter
2 tablespoons sunflower oil
4 teaspoons soy sauce
a good pinch of chilli powder or cayenne pepper
freshly ground black pepper

Prepare the pineapple and cut into small chunks. Reserve 4 tablespoons of the juice.

Rinse and drain the bean sprouts. Discard any discoloured parts and pat dry. Peel and coarsely grate the carrots. Cut the cucumber into sticks. Trim the spring onions and slice diagonally. Reserve about one-third of the peanuts for garnish and combine the remainder with the other salad ingredients in a large bowl.

Whisk the peanut butter into the pineapple juice, add

the oil and soy sauce. Add the chilli powder or cayenne, and season to taste with pepper.

Add the dressing to the salad and toss. Garnish with the reserved peanuts and serve at room temperature.

Monkfish with a Trio of Vegetables

Serves 4
330 calories per serving
Wine suggestion: Riesling

450g monkfish tails
salt and 1 tablespoon coarsely crushed black peppercorns
1 tablespoon extra virgin olive oil
15g unsalted butter
150ml fish stock
1 teaspoon arrowroot
4 tablespoons single cream
2 tablespoons brandy
3 carrots, peeled and cut into ribbons
3 courgettes, washed and cut into ribbons
watercress to garnish

Skin the tails and remove the pink membranes. Cut down either side of the central bone to remove the fillets. Gently rub a little salt and the crushed peppercorns into the fish and sauté for about 10 minutes. Remove the fish.

Mix the arrowroot with a little water to make a paste and stir into the sauce. Add the cream and the brandy, and stir for a few minutes until slightly thickened. Replace the fish.

Cook the vegetables in a little lightly salted water until tender. Serve the fish garnished with the vegetables and watercress.

Beef and Beer Casserole

Serves 4
330 calories per serving
Wine suggestion: Pinot Gris

450g lean stewing steak, in one piece
2 teaspoons margarine
1 medium onion, chopped
1 large carrot, chopped
1 large swede, chopped
240g parsnips, chopped
180g celeriac or celery, trimmed and sliced
300ml beer
600ml beef stock
1 tablespoon Worcestershire sauce
1 tablespoon cornflour, blended with a little water
salt and freshly ground black pepper

Preheat the oven to 150°C/Gas 2. Place the steak on the rack of a grill pan and grill until the fat stops dripping, turning once. Cool slightly and cut into 2.5cm pieces.

Heat the margarine in a large flameproof casserole dish. Add the onion and sauté gently for 10–15 minutes.

Add the vegetables to the casserole together with the beef, beer and stock. Stir in the Worcestershire sauce. Season well. Cook for 1½–2 hours until the meat is tender. Add the blended cornflour stirring until thickened. Cook for 2 more minutes, then taste and adjust the seasoning. Serve hot with a green vegetable.

Seafood Pancakes with a Piquant Sauce

Serves 2
330 calories per serving
Wine suggestion: Chardonnay

60g plain flour
¼ teaspoon salt
1 small egg
150ml skimmed milk
2 teaspoons parsley or chives, finely chopped
1 Cal spray
225g mixed seafood (smoked fish, crab, prawns)
1 small onion, finely chopped
75ml fish stock
1 tablespoon plain flour
150ml skimmed milk
½ teaspoon mustard
dash of Tabasco sauce
½ teaspoon dried mixed herbs
salt and freshly ground black pepper

Preheat the oven to 190°C/Gas 5. Sift the flour and salt into a bowl. Add the egg and a little milk, and stir into the flour to make a thick paste. Gradually add the remaining milk and the herbs. Whisk to a smooth consistency and put to one side.

Prepare the fish and remove any bones.

Dry-fry the onion in a non-stick pan until soft. Add 1 tablespoon of the fish stock and the flour, and cook for about a minute, stirring well. Gradually add the remaining stock and milk, stirring continuously to remove any lumps. Bring to the boil and allow to thicken. Stir in the mustard, Tabasco and mixed herbs, and season well with salt and black pepper. Add half the sauce to the seafood mixture and fold in carefully.

Spray a non-stick pan with the 1 Cal oil. Beat the batter well. Add 2 tablespoons to the hot pan and allow the batter to coat the base of the pan. Cook quickly for about 20 seconds, then flip over and cook the other side. Slide on to a plate. Repeat until you have 4 pancakes.

Divide the fish mixture between the pancakes, fold over and place in a sprayed ovenproof dish. Spoon the remaining sauce over the top and bake in the oven for about 25 minutes.

Brown Rice Paella

Serves 4
345 calories per serving
Wine suggestion: Pinot Gris

360g skinless chicken
1 Cal spray
180g onion, chopped
1 large garlic clove, chopped
180g tomatoes, skinned, seeded and diced
180g red pepper, seeded and chopped
570ml chicken stock
½ teaspoon ground turmeric
1 teaspoon paprika
270g long-grain brown rice (easy cook)
120g frozen peas
200g peeled prawns
salt and freshly ground black pepper

Spray a non-stick pan with 1 Cal oil, then sauté the chicken until golden on both sides and put to one side. Reduce the heat, add the onions and garlic and cook gently for 5 minutes. Add the tomatoes and pepper and cook for a further 3 minutes, stirring constantly. Add the stock and bring to the boil. Replace the chicken and cook over a moderate heat for about 20 minutes. Add the paprika, peas and the rice and stir. Now cook without stirring until all the liquid has been absorbed and the rice is cooked. Add the prawns to the rice mixture and cook for 2 minutes. Season and serve.

Seaside Fish Cakes

Serves 4
345 calories per serving
Wine suggestion: Gewurztraminer

575g potatoes
115g fresh or tinned crab
2 tablespoons fresh chives
juice of ½ lemon
1 teaspoon Worcestershire sauce
3–4 drops chilli sauce
2 eggs, separated
2 tablespoons wholemeal flour
115g fresh wholemeal breadcrumbs
1 tablespoon olive oil
salt and freshly ground black pepper

Preheat the oven to 220°C/Gas 7. Cook the potatoes in salted boiling water for 10–15 minutes until tender. Drain and return to the pan, cooking over a gentle heat to evaporate as much water as possible. Mash well and put into a bowl. Add the crabmeat, chives, lemon juice and chilli sauce and season to taste with salt. Bind the mixture together with the egg yolks.

Refrigerate the mixture for about 1 hour before shaping it into 4 equal cakes. Put the seasoned flour and breadcrumbs on separate flat plates. Lightly whip the egg whites and mix in ¼ teaspoon of salt and a good grinding of pepper. Dip the cakes in the flour, then the egg white and finally the breadcrumbs.

Place the cakes on a non-stick baking tray and sprinkle over the oil. Bake in the oven for about 15 minutes until crisp and golden. Dish up the crab cakes and garnish with the lemon wedges and watercress. Serve with a large green salad and a calorie-free dressing – sushi vinegar would be very tasty.

Wild Rice, Orange and Hazelnut Salad

Serves 6
350 calories per serving
Wine suggestion: Chardonnay

225g wild rice
1 teaspoon salt
juice and grated zest of 1 orange
75g hazelnuts
4 tablespoons currants
1 fennel bulb
1 apple
salt and freshly ground black pepper

For the dressing
3 spring onions
4 tablespoons lemon juice
1 teaspoon balsamic or cider vinegar
1 tablespoon fresh parsley, chopped
1 tablespoon fresh fennel leaves, chopped
¼ teaspoon crushed fennel seeds
3 tablespoons extra virgin olive oil
1 tablespoon hazelnut oil

Preheat the oven to 180°C/Gas 4. Rinse the wild rice and soak for 45 minutes and drain. Bring 1.4 litres of water to the boil with ½ teaspoon of salt, add the rice, cover and simmer for 30 minutes until tender. Drain and set aside.

Roast the hazelnuts on a baking tray in the oven for

6–8 minutes. Place the currants in a bowl, cover with hot water and soak for 5 minutes. Drain and cover with orange juice. Cool the roasted nuts, rub away the skins in a cloth and chop roughly.

Finely chop the spring onion bulbs and roughly chop about 1 tablespoon of the green parts. Mix with the grated orange zest, lemon juice, parsley, vinegar, remaining salt, fennel leaves and seeds and oils. Drain the orange juice from the currants.

Slice the fennel finely, core and dice the apple, and stir into the rice with the currants. Mix well with 1 tablespoon of the dressing. Before serving, add the remaining dressing and nuts. Season and toss well.

Cheesy Jacket Potatoes

Serves 4
350 calories per serving
Wine suggestion: Riesling

4 x 240g baking potatoes, scrubbed
2 spring onions, finely chopped
120g mature Cheddar cheese, grated
2 tablespoons skimmed milk
2 eggs, separated
salt and freshly ground black pepper
few drops of Worcestershire sauce

Preheat the oven to 200°C/Gas 6. Bake the potatoes for approximately 1 hour until just tender. Halve them and scoop out the flesh into a mixing bowl. Reserve the skins. Mash the potato and mix in the spring onions, half the cheese, the milk and egg yolks. Season with salt, pepper and a few drops of Worcestershire sauce.

Whisk the egg whites in a grease-free bowl until stiff. Fold them into the potato mixture, then pile this filling back into the potato skins. Place in a shallow ovenproof dish and sprinkle with the reserved cheese.

Return the potatoes to the oven and bake for a further 15–20 minutes until golden brown. Serve at once with a large green salad.

Lunch Box Humous with Crudités

Serves 2
350 calories per serving
Wine suggestion: Chardonnay

400g can chickpeas, drained and rinsed
1 or 2 large garlic cloves, crushed
1 bunch fresh coriander or parsley
juice and zest of 1 small lemon
4 tablespoons light olive oil
salt and freshly ground black pepper

For dipping
2 mini pitta breads, toasted
2 medium carrots, cut into batons
½ cucumber, cut into batons
6 cherry tomatoes
2 celery sticks, cut into chunks

Process the chickpeas, garlic and herbs together with the zest and lemon juice. With the motor running, add the olive oil until you have a smooth paste. Season with the salt and pepper.

Spicy Lamb and Lentils

Serves 4
355 calories per serving
Wine suggestion: Chenin Blanc

450g lean lamb, trimmed and cut into 25mm dice
1 large onion, finely sliced
2 large garlic cloves, finely sliced
2 large carrots, sliced into thick batons
400g tin tomatoes
1 teaspoon chilli sauce
225g lentils
lamb or vegetable stock
½ teaspoon cumin powder
½ teaspoon ground coriander
450g spinach, well washed
2 tablespoons parsley, chopped
salt and freshly ground black pepper

If the lentils need soaking, do so overnight.

Heat a non-stick casserole pan until it is hot, but not too hot. Put in the lamb (it should sizzle on contact with the hot pan). Move the meat around the pan with a wooden palette until it is sealed and brown. Remove from the pan and wipe away any fat that may have come out of the meat.

Add the onion, garlic and carrots to the pan, and cook over a moderate heat until softened. Now add the tomatoes, lamb, chilli sauce and lentils. Pour in enough stock to cover. Stir in the spices and simmer for about an hour until the meat and vegetables are tender. You may add a little more stock if the mixture becomes too dry.

In the meantime, wash the spinach and wilt quickly in a pan with just the water remaining on the leaves from washing. Stir the spinach into the casserole and sprinkle with chopped parsley.

Spicy Chicken with Dried Fruits and Colourful Peppers

Serves 4
360 calories per serving
Wine suggestion: Sauvignon Blanc

285ml chicken stock
150ml fresh orange juice
2 teaspoons paprika
2 teaspoons ground ginger
½ teaspoon ground cinnamon
½ teaspoon ground allspice
250g ready-to-eat dried fruit salad
4 x 275g skinless chicken thighs (with bones)
salt and freshly ground black pepper

For the peppers
40g butter
3 tablespoons water
4 leeks, washed and thinly sliced
1 tablespoon extra virgin olive oil
2 yellow peppers, seeded and sliced into strips
1 red pepper, seeded and sliced into strips
1½ tablespoons fresh mixed herbs
salt and freshly ground black pepper

Pour the chicken stock and the orange juice into a flameproof casserole dish, then add the spices and stir well. Add the dried fruit and slowly bring to the boil, stirring continuously. Add the chicken and season to taste. Baste the chicken well with the liquid. Lower the heat and cover the pan with a tightly fitting lid. Simmer very gently for about 30 minutes until the chicken is tender. Lift the lid occasionally during cooking, and stir to ensure even cooking. Adjust the seasoning.

Melt the butter in a pan with the water and add the leeks with a little salt. Cover the pan and cook over a medium heat for 8 minutes until tender. Uncover the pan, add the oil and raise the heat. Sauté the peppers for 2 minutes. Add a little more water, lower the heat and cook for a further 2 minutes until the peppers are soft and there is a sweet sauce in the pan. Add the herbs, season and serve.

Salmon and Broccoli Crumble

Serves 4
375 calories per serving
Wine suggestion: Chenin Blanc

90g plain flour
30g rolled oats
1 teaspoon dried mixed herbs
45g margarine
180g broccoli, broken into small florets
60g cornflour
300ml skimmed milk
300ml vegetable stock
1 tablespoon fresh dill, chopped,
    or 1½ teaspoons dried
1 tablespoon fresh parsley, chopped,
    or 1½ teaspoons dried
210g tinned red salmon
salt and freshly ground black pepper

Preheat the oven to 200°C/Gas 6. Sift the flour into a large bowl and mix in the rolled oats, a pinch of salt and the dried mixed herbs. Rub in the margarine until the mixture resembles fine breadcrumbs. Cook the broccoli in lightly salted boiling water until tender – about 5 minutes. Drain well.

In a large jug, blend the cornflour with 5 tablespoons of the milk. Heat the remaining milk in a saucepan with the stock, dill and parsley. When almost boiling, pour on to the blended cornflour, stirring continuously. Return to the saucepan and heat gently, stirring until smooth and thickened.

Drain any liquid from the tinned salmon into the herb sauce. Remove any skin and bone from the salmon, and break into chunks. Add the broccoli to the sauce and stir through. Season with salt and pepper. Pour into an ovenproof baking dish and scatter the salmon chunks on top. Stir them in gently so that they are covered with sauce.

Sprinkle the crumble mixture evenly over the surface and bake in the oven for 20–30 minutes.

Mediterranean Pitta Rounds

Serves 8
380 calories per serving
Wine suggestion: Sauvignon Blanc

2 x 410g tinned chickpeas
60ml skimmed milk
60ml fresh lemon juice
5 garlic cloves
8 x 20cm pitta bread rounds
1 teaspoon olive oil
300g frozen, chopped spinach, thawed and drained
360g tomato, chopped
180g green pepper, diced
180g red pepper, diced
240g crumbled feta cheese
90g olives, sliced

Preheat the oven to 230°C/Gas 8. Blend the first four ingredients in a food processor until smooth. Set aside.

Arrange the pitta rounds on non-stick baking sheets, brush with olive oil and bake for 6 minutes.

Spread the chickpea mixture evenly over the pittas, leaving a small border. Arrange the spinach and the remaining ingredients evenly on top. Bake again for 5 minutes or until they are thoroughly heated and the crust is crisp.

Irish Stew

Serves 4
390 calories per serving
Wine suggestion: Pinot Gris

450g lean neck of lamb fillet
900g potatoes, peeled and thinly sliced
2 large onions, sliced into rings
2 teaspoons fresh rosemary, chopped,
  or 1 teaspoon dried
2 teaspoons fresh thyme, chopped,
  or 1 teaspoon dried
lamb stock
salt and freshly ground black pepper
chopped parsley to garnish

Preheat the oven to 180°C/Gas 4. Cut the meat into thin slices, trimming away any fat. Line the bottom of a casserole dish with a layer of potatoes, then a layer of onion rings and a layer of lamb. Sprinkle with a little rosemary and thyme, and season. Continue layering the meat, vegetables and herbs, finishing with a layer of potato.

Pour in enough stock to half fill the casserole dish and slowly bring to the boil. Cover with foil and the casserole lid, and cook in the oven for about 2½ hours until the potatoes and lamb are tender. Uncover the casserole for the last 20 minutes to brown the potatoes. Garnish with the chopped parsley.

Fruits of the Vine with Rice

Serves 4
390 calories per serving
Wine suggestion: Semillon

30g sultanas
30g raisins
180g brown rice
1 bunch spring onions, finely chopped
135g seedless grapes, halved
90g Red Leicester cheese, cut into small cubes
30g salted roast peanuts
60ml orange juice
2 tablespoons cider vinegar
2 teaspoons olive oil
1 tablespoon mint, chopped
salt and freshly ground black pepper
mint or basil leaves to garnish

Cover the sultanas and raisins with boiling water. Leave
to soak for about 30 minutes. Cook the brown rice until
just tender. Rinse, drain and transfer to a bowl. Drain the
dried fruit and mix with the rice. Add the spring onions,
grapes, cheese and peanuts. Season with salt and pepper.

Mix together the orange juice, vinegar, olive oil and
mint. Season and toss with the salad. Garnish with the
herbs and serve.

Lamb and Potato Moussaka

Serves 4
395 calories per serving
Wine suggestion: Pinot Gris

480g potatoes
1 medium aubergine, sliced
240g lean minced lamb
1 teaspoon margarine
30g plain flour
1 teaspoon paprika
4 teaspoons olive oil
1 garlic clove, crushed
1 medium onion, chopped
240g mushrooms, sliced
150ml vegetable stock
1 teaspoon dried oregano
1 egg
150ml low-fat natural yogurt
60g mature Cheddar cheese, grated

Preheat the oven to 190°C/Gas 5. Cook the potatoes in plenty of lightly salted water until barely tender. Cool and slice. Spread out the aubergine slices and sprinkle liberally with salt to extract the bitter juices. Leave for 10–15 minutes, then turn them over and repeat. Rinse well, but do not pat dry.

Form the minced lamb into small patties and grill until the fat stops dripping, turning once.

Grease a shallow ovenproof baking dish with the margarine. Sprinkle the flour and paprika on to a plate. Lightly coat the aubergine in this seasoned flour and then sauté in 2 teaspoons of the oil for about 1 minute each side. Line the baking dish with the lightly cooked aubergine slices.

Heat the remaining oil and sauté the garlic, onion and mushrooms for 3–4 minutes. Crumble in the lamb and then add the stock and oregano. Cook for 10 minutes, uncovered. Spoon into the baking dish and season with salt and pepper. Arrange the sliced potato on top.

Beat the egg and yogurt together and spread on top of the potatoes. Sprinkle with the cheese and bake for 30–35 minutes until golden brown.

The White Wine Diet Recipes

RECIPES UNDER 500 CALORIES

Ham in Cider

Serves 8
400 calories per serving
Wine suggestion: Chardonnay

1.4kg gammon joint
1 teaspoon ground mace
1 teaspoon ground allspice
12 cloves
570ml dry cider
1 tablespoon sage, thyme or parsley,
chopped grated rind and strained juice
  of ½ an orange and ½ a lemon
225g redcurrant jelly
1 large glass port or red wine
pinch of cayenne pepper
1 tablespoon Worcestershire sauce

Soak the ham overnight in cold water.

Put the ham in a large pan with a tightly fitting lid, together with the cider, spices and herbs. Pour in enough hot water to cover the ham and bring to the boil. Reduce the heat and simmer for 1¼ hours.

To make the sauce, first heat the jelly in a small pan. Add the port and bring gently to the boil, stirring frequently. Reduce the heat and simmer until the liquid has thickened and reduced by about one-third. Stir in the orange and lemon rinds and juice, add the cayenne pepper and the Worcestershire sauce, and mix well. The sauce can be served warm or cold. Drain the ham well and place on a carving dish. Remove all visible fat before carving.

Chicken Cassoulet

Serves 4
400 calories per serving
Wine suggestion: Chenin Blanc

1 tablespoon olive oil
180g baby onions, peeled
1 large garlic clove, crushed
1 large carrot, sliced
180g green beans, sliced
180g mangetout, trimmed
240g new potatoes, scrubbed
420g tin haricot beans, rinsed and drained
900ml vegetable stock
8 x 75g skinned chicken thighs
3 tablespoons fresh herbs, chopped
1 tablespoon cornflour, blended with a little water
salt and freshly ground black pepper

Preheat the oven to 170°C/Gas 3. Heat the oil in a flameproof casserole dish. Sauté the onions, garlic and carrot for 3–4 minutes. Remove from the heat. Add the green beans, mangetout, potatoes, haricot beans, stock and chicken to the casserole. Stir in 2 tablespoons of chopped herbs and season. Cover and cook in the oven for 1¼ hours until the vegetables are cooked and the chicken is very tender. Stir in the blended cornflour and cook for 2–3 minutes until thickened. Serve the cassoulet into 4 warmed bowls and sprinkle with the remaining herbs.

Cheese, Onion and Potato Pie

Serves 4
400 calories per serving
Wine suggestion: Chenin Blanc

960g potatoes, peeled and cut into chunks
2 large onions, sliced
150g mature Cheddar cheese, grated
1 tablespoon fresh chives or parsley, chopped,
   or 1½ teaspoons dried
1 teaspoon margarine
1 egg
150ml low-fat natural yogurt
pinch of nutmeg
salt and freshly ground black pepper

Preheat the oven to 200°C/Gas 6. Cook the potatoes and
onions in a large saucepan of lightly salted water for about
15 minutes until just tender. Drain well and then add
approximately two-thirds of the cheese, stirring to melt.
Season with salt and pepper and mix in the herbs.

Grease an ovenproof baking dish with the margarine,
then spoon in the mixture. Beat together the egg, yogurt
and nutmeg, and spread in an even layer over the surface.
Sprinkle the reserved cheese on top.

Bake for 20–25 minutes until set and golden brown.
Serve with a crisp salad or some lightly steamed green
vegetables.

Ham Salad with a Difference

Serves 4
410 calories per serving
Wine suggestion: Chenin Blanc

1kg new potatoes, halved if large
175g feta cubes in oil
1 teaspoon dried oregano
8 tomatoes, skinned and roughly chopped
100g pitted black olives
200g thick-sliced lean ham, cut into large pieces
2 tablespoons chopped parsley

Bring a large pan of water to the boil. Add the potatoes and cook for 15 minutes until tender.

Heat 2 tablespoons of the feta oil in a pan. Add the oregano and tomatoes and cook for 3–4 minutes until slightly softened. Mix in the olives, feta cubes and ham, and stir well. Drain the potatoes and return to the pan

Tip the ham mixture into the potato pan and season. Toss and sprinkle over the parsley. Serve warm or cold.

Chicken and Vegetable Casserole

Serves 8
415 calories per serving
Wine suggestion: Gewurztraminer

2 tablespoons olive oil
25g butter
8 large skinless, boneless chicken breasts,
   each cut into 3 pieces
8 shallots, peeled and halved
2 garlic cloves, chopped
450g new potatoes, halved
450g baby carrots, scrubbed
3 tablespoons plain flour
1½ tablespoons Dijon mustard
425ml dry white wine
425ml chicken stock
225g asparagus tips, trimmed
225g shelled, fresh or frozen broad beans
   (thaw if frozen)
1 tablespoon lemon juice
100ml double cream
3 or 4 tablespoons parsley and tarragon, chopped

Heat the oil and butter in a large pan and cook the chicken
in batches for 3–4 minutes until golden all over. Remove
from the pan and set aside. Add the shallots, garlic,
potatoes and carrots and toss together. Cook for about 5
minutes until they begin to turn golden. Sprinkle with the

flour, stir in the mustard and toss well. Pour over the wine and gently simmer until reduced by about half.

Pour in the stock, bring to a simmer and return the chicken to the pan. Cover and simmer for about 15 minutes.

Scatter over the asparagus and broad beans without stirring, then cover and simmer for a further 8 minutes. Stir in the lemon juice, cream, parsley and tarragon, and heat through gently. Transfer to a warm serving dish and serve.

Sardine and Tomato Pizza

Serves 4
420 calories per serving
Wine suggestion: Riesling

180g plain flour
45g margarine
1 tablespoon tomato purée
1 teaspoon olive oil
1 small onion, finely chopped
60g mature Cheddar cheese, grated
120g tinned sardines in tomato sauce
4 medium tomatoes, sliced
2 teaspoons dried oregano
salt and freshly ground black pepper
parsley to garnish

Preheat the oven to 200°C/Gas 6. Sift the flour and a pinch of salt into a large bowl. Rub in the margarine until the mixture resembles fine breadcrumbs, and add sufficient cold water to make a soft dough. Knead lightly until smooth. On a lightly floured surface, roll out to a circle approximately 25cm in diameter. Lift on to a baking sheet and brush with tomato purée. Heat the oil in a small frying pan and sauté the onion until softened. Scatter evenly over the pizza base with most of the cheese. Arrange the sardines and sliced tomatoes on top, and season. Sprinkle with the oregano and remaining cheese. Bake for about 25 minutes. Slice into 4 portions and serve with a green salad.

Orange-Roasted Fennel and Bulgar Wheat Salad

Serves 4
420 calories per serving
Wine suggestion: Chardonnay

250g bulgar wheat
1 litre boiling water
3 heads of fennel, cut into wedges
4 tablespoons olive oil
zest and juice of 2 oranges
4 tablespoons fresh flatleaf parsley
2 tablespoons fresh mint, chopped
4 plum tomatoes, cut into wedges
140g mixed olives, drained
100g rocket

Preheat the oven to 180°C/Gas 4. Place the bulgar wheat in a large bowl and cover with the boiling water and allow to stand for 30 minutes. Place the fennel in a large roasting tin, drizzle with the olive oil and season. Add the orange zest and half the orange juice, and roast in the oven for 35 minutes until softened and slightly charred.

Drain the bulgar wheat, then add the parsley, mint and remaining orange juice. Combine well and season to taste. Place the tomatoes, olives and rocket in a large bowl. Add the roasted fennel with the pan juices and toss well. Divide the bulgar wheat between 4 serving plates, top with the fennel and tomato mixture, and serve.

American Baked Beans

Serves 4
420 calories per serving
Wine suggestion: Pinot Gris

240g lean pork shoulder, in one piece
120g pork and beef sausage, twisted and snipped in half
2 teaspoons vegetable oil
1 large onion, chopped
1 medium apple, peeled, cored and chopped
1 carrot, sliced
420g tinned tomatoes
540g tinned borlotti beans, rinsed and drained
600ml vegetable stock
2 tablespoons tomato purée
½ teaspoon ground ginger
1 tablespoon molasses sugar
1 tablespoon cornflour, blended with a little water
salt and freshly ground black pepper
chopped fresh thyme or parsley to garnish

Preheat the oven to 150°C/Gas 2. Place the pork and sausages on a grill rack. Grill until the fat stops dripping, turning the pork once and the sausages until they are browned all over.

Heat the oil in a large flameproof casserole dish and sauté the onion, apple and carrot for about 5 minutes until softened. Cut the pork into 2.5cm pieces and add to the casserole with the sausages, tomatoes, beans, stock,

128

tomato purée, ginger and molasses sugar. Stir well and season with salt and pepper.

Cover and cook in the oven for about 1½ hours or until the pork is tender. Add the blended cornflour and stir until thickened. Cook for 2 minutes and then ladle into warmed serving bowls. Sprinkle with chopped herbs and serve at once.

White Fish and Cheddar Lasagne

Serves 4
430 calories per serving
Wine suggestion: Semillon

2 teaspoons olive oil
1 small onion, finely chopped
120g button mushrooms, sliced
420g tinned tomatoes, chopped
1 small courgette, sliced
150ml vegetable stock
1 tablespoon margarine
30g plain flour
300ml skimmed milk
120g mature Cheddar cheese, grated
1 tablespoon fresh marjoram or parsley, chopped
120g (6 sheets) precooked spinach lasagne
360g white fish, skinned, boned and cut into chunks
salt and freshly ground black pepper

Preheat the oven to 190°C/Gas 5. Heat the oil in a saucepan and sauté the onion and mushrooms for about 5 minutes. Add the tomatoes, courgette and stock, then simmer, uncovered, for 15–20 minutes until reduced. Season to taste.

Put the margarine, flour and milk into a small saucepan and heat, whisking constantly until the sauce boils and thickens. Remove from the heat and add half the cheese and the herbs. Stir gently to melt the cheese and season to taste.

Spoon the tomato mixture into a greased shallow baking dish and top with half the lasagne sheets. Scatter the fish over the top, then pour over half the cheese sauce. Top with the remaining lasagne sheets and spread the rest of the cheese sauce on top. Sprinkle with the remaining cheese.

Cover with foil and bake for 20 minutes. Remove the foil and cook for a further 20 minutes.

Fish and Chickpea Curry

Serves 4
455 calories per serving
Wine suggestion: Semillon

1 tablespoon margarine
1 medium apple, peeled, cored and chopped
1 large onion, chopped
2 tablespoons curry powder
600ml vegetable stock
420g tinned tomatoes, chopped
2 tablespoons tomato purée
30g sultanas
540g tinned chickpeas, rinsed and drained
120g long-grain rice
480g white fish, skinned, boned and cut into chunks
1 tablespoon chopped coriander or parsley
4 tablespoons low-fat natural yogurt
salt and freshly ground black pepper
herbs to garnish

Melt the margarine in a large saucepan and sauté the apple and onion for 3–4 minutes. Add the curry powder and cook gently, stirring for 2 minutes. Add the vegetable stock, tomatoes, purée, sultanas and chickpeas. Season with salt and pepper, then simmer gently, covered, for 30 minutes

Cook the rice in lightly salted boiling water for about 12 minutes.

Add the fish to the curry in the pan but do not stir.

Replace the lid and cook for 5–8 minutes until the fish looks opaque and flakes easily.

Drain the rice well, rinse with boiling water and allow to drain thoroughly. Spoon equal quantities of rice on to 4 plates. Add the chopped herbs to the curry and stir gently to avoid breaking up the pieces of fish, then ladle on to the plates. Garnish with a tablespoon of yogurt and fresh herbs.

Spaghetti Surprise

Serves 4
465 calories per serving
Wine suggestion: Pinot Gris

30g pine nuts
240g spaghetti
2 large courgettes, sliced
240g low-fat soft cheese
150ml skimmed milk
1 tablespoon oregano, chopped, or 1½ teaspoons dried
60g blue cheese, crumbled
salt and freshly ground black pepper

Toast the pine nuts under a preheated grill until golden. Set aside. Cook the spaghetti in a large saucepan of lightly salted water for 6–8 minutes until just tender. Meanwhile, simmer the courgettes in a small amount of lightly salted water for about 5 minutes.

Gently heat the soft cheese and milk in a small pan until almost boiling, stirring constantly. Season with salt and pepper and stir in the oregano.

Drain the spaghetti and courgettes, then toss together. Add the sauce, blue cheese and pine nuts, and stir together gently until thoroughly combined. Divide the food between 4 warmed plates and serve hot.

Chicken Salad

Serves 4
475 calories per serving
Wine suggestion: Sauvignon Blanc

1 cos lettuce
2 skinless, boneless chicken breasts
7 tablespoons olive oil
1 small French loaf
2 garlic cloves, finely chopped
50g Parmesan cheese, finely grated
salt and freshly ground black pepper

For the dressing
2 tablespoons lemon juice
1 teaspoon Worcestershire sauce
1 tablespoon mayonnaise

Preheat the oven to 170°C/Gas 3. Wash and dry the lettuce, tear the leaves into large pieces and chill in a large polythene bag to crisp them up. Preheat a griddle pan. Bat out the chicken breasts and brush with 1 tablespoon of the olive oil. Season. Griddle on each side until cooked.

Cut the French bread into large cubes and toss in half the garlic and 2 tablespoons of the oil. Spread over a baking sheet and bake the croutons for 10–15 minutes until crisp.

Tip the lettuce into a large serving bowl and sprinkle over half the Parmesan and all the croutons. Put the remaining oil, garlic, lemon juice, Worcestershire sauce and seasoning in a screw-topped jar. Shake the jar well to mix, then add the mayonnaise to the jar and shake again.

Cut the chicken into strips and add to the salad. Toss the dressing into the salad, sprinkle with the reserved Parmesan and serve.

Ham and Pea Risotto

Serves 4
495 calories per serving
Wine suggestion: Sauvignon Blanc

4 thin slices lean cooked ham, cut into strips
2 tablespoons olive oil
15g butter
1 medium onion, finely chopped
350g short-grain risotto rice
150ml dry white wine
1.1 litres vegetable stock
75g frozen peas
50g freshly grated Parmesan cheese
salt and freshly ground black pepper

Heat the oil and butter over a gentle heat and cook the onion until it is soft and golden. Add the rice to the onions and cook over a moderate heat for 5 minutes until the grains begin to burst. Heat the stock. Stir the wine into the rice and cook until it has been absorbed. Add a ladleful of the hot stock. Mix well and continue cooking over a moderate heat until absorbed, stirring continuously.

Continue cooking for a further 20 minutes adding the stock a ladleful at a time until the rice is tender and the texture is creamy. Add the peas with the last measure of stock and season to taste. Fold in the ham and 25g of the Parmesan. Serve, sprinkled with Parmesan.

RECIPES UNDER 900 CALORIES

Indian Chickpea Salad

Serves 4
640 calories per serving
Wine suggestion: Riesling

6 tablespoons olive oil
3 garlic cloves, sliced
2 red chillis, halved, seeded and sliced
4 teaspoons cumin seeds, lightly crushed
2 x 400g tins chickpeas, drained and rinsed
3 tomatoes, halved, seeded and diced
zest and juice of 1 lemon
1 naan bread

For the salad
25g fresh coriander
½ cucumber, cut into thick batons
1 medium red onion, thinly sliced
100g fresh baby spinach

Put 5 tablespoons of the oil into a large pan and add the garlic, chillis and cumin. Warm over a medium heat for 10 minutes ensuring that the garlic doesn't burn. Add the chickpeas and warm through for 5 minutes.

Meanwhile, preheat the grill to high. Add the tomatoes, lemon zest and juice to the chickpeas and season. Set aside this mixture. Brush the naan with remaining oil and grill both sides until crisp and golden. Tear into 3cm pieces.

Toss together the salad ingredients and divide between 4 plates. Spoon the chickpea mixture over and top with the naan croutons.

One-Pot Roasted Lamb with Summer Vegetables

Serves 6
675 calories per serving
Wine suggestion: Chardonnay

900g lean boneless lamb shoulder, fillet or leg
900g new potatoes, halved if large
4 courgettes
6 large ripe tomatoes, skinned
6 garlic cloves
285g jar artichoke hearts in oil, drained,
    reserving 2 tablespoons of the oil
2 tablespoons olive oil
175ml dry white wine

For the mint pesto
2 tablespoons toasted flaked almonds
large bunch of fresh mint, stalks removed
1 teaspoon Dijon mustard
juice of ½ lemon
6 tablespoons olive oil

Preheat the oven to 170°C/Gas 3. Cut the lamb into 5cm chunks. Parboil the potatoes. Cut the courgettes into 5cm chunks, quarter the tomatoes, peel and slice the garlic cloves. Mix together the lamb, potatoes, courgettes, tomatoes, garlic, artichokes, oil and salt and pepper in a roasting tin, then spread out.

Bake for 45–55 minutes until the lamb is browned and

tender and the vegetables are cooked. Splash in the white wine halfway through cooking and stir gently.

To make the pesto, put the almonds in a food processor and process until chopped. Add the mint, mustard and lemon and process to a rough paste. Gradually add the oil and season well. Spoon the pesto into a small bowl and serve separately with the lamb.

Club Sandwich

Serves 2
690 calories per serving
Wine suggestion: Chardonnay

60g low-fat spread
12 slices wholemeal bread
1 medium carrot, grated
60g bean sprouts
60g iceberg lettuce, shredded
½ teaspoon poppy seeds
1 tablespoon lemon juice
1 tablespoon cider vinegar
1 teaspoon wholegrain mustard
120g lean ham or chicken
120g tomatoes, sliced
salt and freshly ground black pepper

Spread a little low-fat spread on each slice of bread. Mix together the carrot, bean sprouts, lettuce and poppy seeds. In a small jug, combine the lemon juice, vinegar and mustard, stirring well. Season with a little salt and pepper and then add to the salad mixture.

Make 4 club sandwiches using a generous amount of the salad mixture on the first layer. Cover with a slice of bread and top with the ham or chicken and sliced tomatoes. Season with salt and pepper, then top with the remaining bread.

Fish and Vegetable Pie

Serves 2
690 calories per serving
Wine suggestion: Riesling

720g potatoes, peeled and cut into chunks
480g skinned and boned white fish, such as cod,
   haddock or whiting
1 tablespoon margarine
1 small onion, finely chopped
120g mushrooms, sliced
30g plain flour
450ml skimmed milk
60g frozen peas
45g frozen sweetcorn kernels
1 tablespoon chopped parsley
salt and freshly ground black pepper

Preheat the oven to 200°C/Gas 6. Cook the potatoes in lightly salted boiling water until tender. Poach the fish in a little water for about 8 minutes until it is opaque and flakes easily. Drain off and reserve the cooking liquid. Flake the fish.

Melt the margarine in a pan and sauté the onion for about 3 minutes. Add the mushrooms and cook for 2 more minutes. Stir in the flour and cook for 1 minute and then gradually add the milk, reserving 4 tablespoons. Heat until the sauce boils and thickens, then add the peas, sweetcorn and parsley. Add the fish and reserved cooking liquid, stirring gently to avoid breaking up the fish. Season to taste and pour into an ovenproof baking dish.

Drain and mash the cooked potatoes, adding the reserved milk. Season and beat until fluffy, then spoon or pipe on top of the fish mixture. Bake for about 20 minutes until heated through and browned on the surface.

Sausage Casserole

Serves 2
700 calories per serving
Wine suggestion: Pinot Gris

360g thin-link pork and beef sausages
2 teaspoons vegetable oil
1 large onion, sliced
2 sticks celery, sliced
1 large carrot, sliced
1 beef stock cube
450ml hot water
1 tablespoon tomato purée
90g mangetout, trimmed
salt and freshly ground black pepper
1 tablespoon cornflour, blended with a little water

Grill the sausages, turning until the fat stops dripping and they are well browned. Wipe the surface fat away with kitchen paper.

Melt the margarine in a large frying pan. Sauté the onion, celery and carrot gently for about 8 minutes until softened.

Dissolve the stock cube in the hot water and mix in the tomato purée. Add to the sautéed vegetables with the sausages and mangetout. Season with salt and pepper, then cover and simmer gently for 20–30 minutes until the vegetables are cooked. Add the blended cornflour, stirring until thickened and smooth. Cook for 1 minute and serve hot.

Tomato and Pepper Pasta with Olives

Serves 2
720 calories per serving
Wine suggestion: Riesling

6 large, ripe tomatoes
2 red peppers
4 cloves garlic
4 rosemary sprigs
225g shell pasta
½ teaspoon caster sugar
16 black olives
1 sprig basil leaves
1 teaspoon marjoram, chopped
1 teaspoon chives, chopped
50g Parmesan cheese, grated
salt and freshly ground black pepper

Preheat the oven to 200°C/Gas 6. Wash and dry the tomatoes and peppers. Cut the peppers in half and remove the seeds, then place them in a roasting tray, cover with 2 of the rosemary sprigs, and roast for about 25 minutes. After 10 minutes add the tomatoes and the garlic (without peeling).

Add the pasta to a pan of boiling salted water. Cook according to the instructions on the packet. Drain, rinse in cold running water and drain again. Put aside.

When cool enough to handle, peel away the pepper and tomato skins and squeeze the garlic cloves from their skins. Place the tomatoes, peppers, sugar and garlic in a liquidiser, and blend to a thick sauce. Season the sauce to taste and stir in the olives.

Mix the pasta with the tomato sauce. Tear the basil leaves and add them to the pasta with most of the marjoram and chives. Garnish with the remaining rosemary sprigs and herbs. Serve the salad cold with the freshly grated Parmesan cheese.

Herring with Warm Potato Salad

Serves 2
750 calories per serving
Wine suggestion: Chenin Blanc

480g potatoes, peeled and cut into chunks
4 x 180g herrings, cleaned and boned
finely grated rind and juice of 1 lemon
2 teaspoons wholegrain mustard
1 teaspoon vinegar
150ml low-fat natural yogurt
5cm piece cucumber
2 tablespoons chives or spring onions, chopped
1 teaspoon ground coriander
salt and freshly ground black pepper
chopped chives and tomato wedges, to garnish

Cook the potatoes in plenty of lightly salted boiling water for about 10 minutes until just tender.

Preheat the grill. Slash the herrings and place on the grill rack. Mix together the lemon rind and juice, mustard and vinegar. Season and brush liberally over the fish. Grill for 6–8 minutes each side, basting from time to time.

Drain the potatoes well and allow the steam to evaporate for a few moments. Mix together the yogurt, cucumber, chives or spring onions and ground coriander. Season, then add to the hot potatoes, stirring gently to mix.

Serve the fish with the warm potato salad garnished with chopped chives and tomato wedges.

Autumn Vegetable Slice

Serves 2
800 calories per serving
Wine suggestion: Chardonnay

4 tablespoons margarine
120g bulgar wheat
1 large carrot, grated
1 large onion, finely chopped
1 tablespoon fresh parsley, chopped
90g Double Gloucester cheese, grated
3 eggs, beaten
150ml skimmed milk
salt and freshly ground black pepper

Preheat the oven to 190°C/Gas 5. Grease a 20cm cake tin with 1 teaspoon of margarine. Put the bulgar wheat in a large mixing bowl and pour boiling water over it. Soak for about 20 minutes until the grains swell.

Meanwhile, heat the remaining margarine in a pan and gently sauté the carrot and onion for about 10 minutes, stirring frequently.

Drain the bulgar wheat well and add the carrot, onion, parsley and seasoning. Mix in the grated cheese. Beat the eggs and milk together and add to the mixture, stirring well to combine.

Transfer the mixture to the prepared cake tin and bake for 35–40 minutes until set and golden brown. Allow to cool slightly, then cut into wedges. Serve with a mixed-leaf salad.

Pasta and Vegetable Salad

Serves 2
880 calories per serving
Wine suggestion: Pinot Gris

350g pasta tubes
1 red onion
1 teaspoon cider vinegar
75g broccoli florets
225g small courgette, trimmed and cut into ½-inch dice
2 stalks celery, trimmed and cut into ½-inch dice
½ cucumber, cut into ½-inch dice
2 small carrots, cut into fine matchsticks
8 cherry tomatoes, cut into halves
3 tablespoons fresh basil leaves
3 tablespoons extra virgin olive oil
50g goat's cheese, crumbled
salt and freshly ground black pepper

Slice the onion thinly and pickle it by placing in a bowl and covering with boiling water for about 30 seconds. Drain and return to the bowl with just enough cider vinegar to cover. Store in the refrigerator for about 3 hours.

Cook the pasta. Blanch the broccoli in boiling, salted water for 2 minutes. Drain and put aside.

Combine all the vegetables and the basil together in a serving bowl. Drain and rinse the pasta, toss with the olive oil and add together with the drained onions to the salad bowl. Season, sprinkle with the goat's cheese and serve.

Desserts

Summer Fruits

Serves 4
70 calories per serving
Wine suggestion: Semillon

225g blueberries
115g cherries
115g raspberries
115g strawberries
4 heaped tablespoons Greek yogurt
2 tablespoons Cassis or Ribena
mint to garnish

Prepare the fruit and arrange on 4 plates. Divide the yogurt between the plates and sprinkle with the Cassis or Ribena. Garnish with the mint.

Fresh Peach with a Raspberry Coulis

Serves 4
75 calories per serving
Wine suggestion: Muscat

4 ripe peaches
1 tablespoon lemon juice
1 tablespoon granulated sugar
1 tablespoon Ribena
1 tablespoon water
225g raspberries (fresh or frozen)
fresh mint to garnish

Put the peaches in a large bowl and pour boiling water over them. Allow to stand for 1 minute, then drain and cool. Peel off their skins and sprinkle with the lemon juice to prevent discoloration.

Melt the sugar in a pan with the Ribena and 1 tablespoon of water. Add the raspberries and allow them to soften. Liquidise and then push through a sieve to remove the seeds. Divide the sauce between 4 plates and place a peach on top. Garnish with the mint. If you prefer, you can remove the stones from the peaches and slice them.

Banana and Raspberry Smoothie

Serves 4
110 calories per serving
Wine suggestion: This is a drink in itself, so have your wine with something else!

120g banana
180g frozen raspberries
mint to garnish

Blend together the banana and the unthawed raspberries in a processor until you have a smooth purée. Pour into 4 small glasses and garnish with the mint.

Hot and Spicy Autumn Fruits

Serves 4
110 calories per serving
Wine suggestion: Pinot Gris

2 medium oranges, scrubbed
480g plums, halved and stoned
1 cinnamon stick, or ½ teaspoon ground cinnamon
1 tablespoon granulated sugar
30g sultanas
120ml orange juice
120ml water
4 tablespoons low-fat yogurt

Pare the zest from the oranges using a potato peeler. Place in a medium-sized saucepan with the plums, cinnamon, sugar, sultanas, orange juice and water. Heat gently and simmer, covered, for about 10 minutes until the plums are tender.

Meanwhile, remove the peel and pith from the oranges and cut the flesh into slices. Add the orange slices to the pan and heat through gently, but avoid breaking up the fruit.

Remove the cinnamon stick, if used, and serve the hot fruit with 1 tablespoon of yogurt per portion.

Fresh Fruit Salad with Stem Ginger

Serves 4
120 calories per serving
Wine suggestion: Chardonnay

50g caster sugar
1 tablespoon Cointreau or other liqueur
1 small pineapple
1 Ogen melon
2 ripe Comice pears
juice of ½ lemon
50g stem ginger
fresh mint to garnish

Place the sugar in a basin with 1 tablespoon of water and very slowly bring to the boil. The sugar needs to dissolve before the water boils. Simmer until the liquid is clear and then add the liqueur. Put to one side.

Cut away the outer skin of the pineapple and slice the flesh into small pieces. Cut the melon into 4 and remove the skin and the seeds. Cut up in the same way as the pineapple. Peel, core and cut the pears into uniform slices. Sprinkle the pear slices with the lemon juice to retain their colour. Finely slice the ginger. Mix all the fruits and the ginger together, and mix with the cooled syrup. Cover with cling film and chill for 1 hour if possible. Garnish with the mint.

Baked Apple with Currants

Serves 1
130 calories per serving
Wine suggestion: Pinot Gris

1 x 85g Bramley apple
25g currants
sweetener to taste
apple juice or white wine

Core the apple and stuff with the currants and sweetener to taste. Moisten with a little apple juice or white wine and either bake in the oven or in the microwave until the apple is soft.

Apple Crisp Slices

Serves 8
135 calories per slice
Wine suggestion: Chardonnay

4 medium apples, peeled
45g brown sugar
60g flour
60g rolled oats
1 teaspoon cinnamon
2 tablespoons softened butter

Preheat the oven to 190°C/Gas 5. Coat a 10cm pan with 1 Cal cooking spray. Quarter, core and thinly slice the apples lengthways, then place them neatly in the pan. Mix together the remaining ingredients and sprinkle over the apples. Bake for about 30 minutes.

Autumn Fool

Serves 4
140 calories per serving
Wine suggestion: Muscat

450g fresh or frozen blackberries
25g custard powder
40g caster sugar
285ml skimmed milk
115g thick Greek yogurt
1 teaspoon icing sugar

Put the custard powder into a bowl. Add 15g of the caster sugar and blend to a smooth paste with 4 tablespoons of the milk. Pour the rest of the milk into a small saucepan, bring to the boil and then stir the boiling milk into the custard powder.

Return this mixture to the pan and bring back to the boil, stirring constantly until the custard has thickened.

Pour the mixture into a bowl and allow to cool a little. Cover with cling film before refrigerating for at least 1 hour.

Reserve 4 blackberries for the garnish and put the rest into a pan with the remaining sugar and cook over a low heat for about 7 minutes until the fruit softens. Press the fruit through a sieve to make a purée.

Whisk the chilled custard until very smooth, then whisk in the yogurt and fold in the purée. Spoon into serving glasses and chill. Garnish with the reserved blackberries, sprinkle with the icing sugar and serve.

Summer Fruit Brûlée

Serves 4
170 calories per serving
Wine suggestion: Chardonnay

120g blueberries
120g raspberries
180g strawberries, hulled and sliced
150g redcurrants
artificial sweetener to taste
360g natural low-fat fromage frais
3 tablespoons demerara sugar

Mix all the fruit together and divide between 4 ramekin dishes. Sprinkle to taste with the sweetener. Spoon the fromage frais over the fruit, smoothing it out to completely cover the surface. Chill for 10 minutes.

Preheat the grill. Place the desserts on a baking tray and sprinkle the demerara sugar over the top. Grill for 3–5 minutes until the sugar melts and bubbles. Serve at once, or chill thoroughly for eating later.

Fruity Semolina

Serves 4
175 calories per serving
Wine suggestion: Chenin Blanc

½ teaspoon margarine
600ml skimmed milk
finely grated rind and juice of 2 medium oranges
60g semolina
30g sultanas
30g caster sugar
pinch of ground nutmeg
1 egg, beaten

Preheat the oven to 190°C/Gas 5. Grease an ovenproof dish with the margarine. Put the milk and orange rind in a saucepan. Sprinkle in the semolina and heat until boiling, stirring constantly. Simmer gently for 2–3 minutes and then stir in the orange juice, sultanas, sugar and nutmeg. Add the egg and mix well.

Transfer to the prepared dish and bake for approximately 30 minutes until lightly browned.

Mocha Mousse

Serves 4
175 calories per serving
Wine suggestion: Muscat

60g plain chocolate, broken into pieces
1 tablespoon instant coffee granules
1 tablespoon caster sugar
4 tablespoons hot water
2 eggs, separated
4 tablespoons whipping cream
4 coffee beans to decorate

Put the chocolate into a medium-sized bowl and place over a saucepan of gently simmering water to melt. Dissolve the instant coffee and sugar in the hot water, then add to the chocolate, stirring until smooth and blended. Remove from the heat and cool slightly.

Beat the egg yolks and stir into the chocolate mixture. Return the bowl to the pan of simmering water and cook the mixture, stirring constantly until slightly thickened. Remove from the heat and cool for about 15 minutes. (To prevent a skin from forming, cover the surface with a circle of dampened greaseproof paper.)

Whip the cream in a chilled bowl until it holds its shape, then spoon half of it into a piping bag fitted with a star nozzle. Place this in the refrigerator. In a grease-free bowl, whisk the egg whites until they hold their shape. Fold through the chocolate mixture with the rest of the whipped cream. Divide between 4 small serving glasses.

Decorate the desserts with piped cream and coffee beans, and chill until ready to serve.

This recipe is not suitable for pregnant women, small children or the elderly.

Raisin Bread Pudding

Serves 4
185 calories per serving
Wine suggestion: Pinot Gris

4 teaspoons low-fat spread
4 x 30g slices of raisin bread
450ml skimmed milk
2 eggs, beaten
1 tablespoon caster sugar
½ teaspoon vanilla extract
pinch of ground nutmeg

Preheat the oven to 180°C/Gas 4. Spread 1 teaspoon of low-fat spread over each slice of raisin bread. Cut each slice into triangles and arrange in an ovenproof baking dish.

Beat together the milk, eggs, sugar and vanilla extract, then strain over the bread. Allow to stand for about 15 minutes. Sprinkle with ground nutmeg. Bake for 30–35 minutes until risen and brown.

Clementine Pudding

Serves 4
230 calories per serving
Wine suggestion: Chardonnay

2 tablespoons margarine
4 tablespoons caster sugar
finely grated rind and juice of 1 medium orange
finely grated rind and juice of 2 limes or 1 lemon
2 eggs, separated
60g self-raising flour
300ml skimmed milk

Preheat the oven to 200°C/Gas 6. Beat the margarine and sugar together until light and fluffy. Add the orange rind and lime or lemon rind, and beat into the mixture with the egg yolks.

Sift the flour into the mixture and stir to mix, then gradually add the milk to make a thin batter. Stir in the orange and lime or lemon juice.

Whisk the egg whites in a grease-free bowl until stiff, then fold them into the pudding mixture. Transfer to an ovenproof baking dish.

Stand the baking dish in a roasting pan half filled with warm water and bake for approximately 45 minutes until brown and springy to the touch.

Fresh Orange Jelly

Serves 4
235 calories per serving
Wine suggestion: Semillon

6 large oranges
340ml water
115g sugar
powdered gelatine as per the recommended
 amounts on the packet
2 tablespoons Cointreau

Squeeze the juice from 5 of the oranges and add the water. Measure the quantity of liquid to work out how much gelatine you will need. Thinly pare the zest from the remaining orange. Put the juice, water and sugar together with the zest in a large pan, and bring slowly to the boil, making sure that the sugar dissolves. Dissolve the gelatine as per the instructions. Remove the zest from the pan. Reduce the heat and stir in the gelatine, then simmer until the gelatine is completely incorporated.

Strain the jelly liquid into a wet mould and stir in the liqueur. Leave in the refrigerator to set for about 2 hours. When set, dip the mould into hot water and upturn on a suitable plate. Decorate the base of the jelly with segments cut from the remaining orange.

Rosy Poached Pears

Serves 4
235 calories per serving
Wine suggestion: Muscat

4 firm dessert pears
285ml red wine
½ glass Cassis or Ribena (optional)
1½ tablespoons lemon juice
1 cinnamon stick or 2 teaspoons ground cinnamon
115g caster sugar
1 tablespoon runny honey
6 cloves
4 bay leaves
twist of freshly ground black pepper
mint sprigs to garnish

Peel the pears and leave them whole with their stalks on. Pour the red wine and optional Cassis into a large pan, then add the lemon juice, cinnamon, sugar, ginger, honey, cloves, bay leaves and black pepper. Heat gently, stirring until the sugar has dissolved.

Add the pears, spoon the mixture over them and cover the pan. Reduce to a low heat and, keeping the liquid just below boiling point, poach gently for about 1 hour, turning occasionally until the pears are soft but still whole. The time they take will be determined by the ripeness of the pears.

Remove the pears from the liquid and arrange on a

serving dish or individual plate. Strain the liquid through a sieve and discard the spices. Reduce the sauce until there is just enough to cover the pears. Coat the pears with the sauce, cover and chill. Garnish with the mint sprigs.

Gooseberry Crumble

Serves 4
240 calories per serving
Wine suggestion: Chardonnay

480g gooseberries, topped and tailed
sweetener to taste
45g plain wholemeal flour
45g rolled oats
pinch of salt
45g margarine
30g soft brown sugar
4 tablespoons low-fat yogurt to serve

Preheat the oven to 200°C/Gas 6. Place the gooseberries in the base of a 1.2-litre ovenproof baking dish, adding sweetener to taste. Add 2 tablespoons of water.

Put the flour, rolled oats and salt into a mixing bowl, and stir well. Rub in the margarine, then stir in the sugar. Sprinkle evenly over the gooseberries. Bake in the oven for 35–40 minutes until golden brown and crunchy on the surface. Serve hot with the yogurt.

Pineapple and Coconut Rum Layer

Serves 4
270 calories per serving
Wine suggestion: Semillon

4 tablespoons whipping cream
2 x 150ml cartons fat-free pineapple yogurt
30g desiccated coconut, toasted
3–4 drops rum essence
470g tin crushed pineapple, drained
4 digestive biscuits, crushed

Whip the cream in a chilled bowl until it holds its shape. Add the yogurt, half the coconut and the rum essence. Fold through gently to mix.

Spoon a layer of crushed pineapple into the base of 4 serving glasses. Sprinkle a layer of biscuit crumbs over the surface, then follow with a layer of the creamy yogurt mixture. Repeat the layers once more, finishing with the cream mixture. Decorate each dessert with the reserved coconut sprinkled on top. Chill before serving.

Cherry Cheesecake

Serves 4
300 calories per serving
Wine suggestion: Muscat

4 digestive biscuits, crushed
360g low-fat soft cheese
150ml fat-free cherry yogurt
1 tablespoon lemon juice
sweetener to taste
180g cherries, halved and stoned
4 tablespoons water
1 teaspoon arrowroot blended with a little water

Sprinkle the biscuit crumbs equally between 4 serving dishes. In a mixing bowl, beat the cheese until soft, then stir in the yogurt and lemon juice. Add sweetener. Fold in one-third of the cherries, then spoon an equal amount of this mixture into each serving dish. Chill.

Put the remaining cherries into a small saucepan with the water. Heat and simmer gently for 2–3 minutes, then stir in the blended arrowroot and cook gently for 1 minute. Cool slightly, then spoon on top of the cheesecakes and chill.

The White Wine Diet Recipes

Individual Chocolate Puddings

Serves 4
315 calories per serving
Wine suggestion: Sauvignon Blanc

45g margarine
45g dark muscovado sugar
2 small eggs, beaten
90g self-raising flour
1 tablespoon warm water
15g chocolate polka dots
1 tablespoon unsweetened cocoa powder
2 tablespoons cornflour
300ml skimmed milk
sweetener to taste

Use ½ teaspoon of margarine to lightly grease 4 small pudding bowls. It might help the turning out of the puddings if you line the base of the bowls or tins with discs of greaseproof paper. Cream the remaining margarine with the sugar until fluffy, then beat in the eggs a little at a time.

Sift the flour into the creamed mixture and fold in with a metal spoon. Add the water to give a soft, dropping consistency and then stir in the chocolate polka dots. Divide this mixture between the prepared bowls so that it comes about two-thirds of the way to the top. Cover with foil.

Transfer the pudding bowls to a steamer and steam for about 40 minutes.

To make the chocolate sauce, mix together the cocoa powder and cornflour, and blend with 5 tablespoons of the milk. Heat the remaining milk until just boiling, then pour on to the blended mixture, stirring constantly. Return to the saucepan and heat gently, stirring, until smooth and thickened. Cool for 1 minute, then add sweetener to taste.

Turn out the puddings and serve with the chocolate sauce.

Surprise Nectarines with a Raspberry Sauce

Serves 4
330 calories per serving
Wine suggestion: Gewurztraminer

180g fresh or frozen raspberries
sweetener to taste
4 very ripe nectarines
¼ lemon
100g cottage cheese
1 tablespoon raisins
2 teaspoons clear honey
sprig of mint

To make the sauce, heat the raspberries gently in a pan, liquidise them and push them through a sieve to remove the seeds. Sweeten if desired and leave to cool. Cut the nectarines in half and remove the stone. Brush the cut edge with lemon juice to prevent discoloration.

Beat the cottage cheese and stir in the chopped raisins and the honey. Mix well. Pile the mixture into the nectarines. Divide the sauce between 4 plates and place 2 nectarine halves on top. Garnish with a sprig of mint.

Bread and Butter Pudding

Serves 4
350 calories per serving
Wine suggestion: Sauvignon Blanc

4 thin slices white bread
50g butter
115g currants
2 eggs and 1 extra yolk
285ml semi-skimmed milk
zest of ½ lemon
1 teaspoon vanilla extract
2 tablespoons runny honey
¼ teaspoon freshly ground nutmeg

Butter the slices of bread and cut each slice into 4 triangles. Grease a 570ml pie dish and arrange the bread in layers, sprinkling each with the currants. Make sure that the final layer is butter-side up.

Beat the eggs together and add the milk. Stir in the lemon rind and the vanilla extract. Pour the liquid over the bread and drizzle the honey over the top. Leave to stand for about 1 hour. Meanwhile, preheat the oven to 180°C/Gas 4.

Sprinkle the top of the pudding with the nutmeg and bake for about 30 minutes or until well risen and golden brown. Serve immediately.

6
Three Weekly Menu Plans for the White Wine Diet

In this chapter you will find three sample weekly menu plans. I have designed them for three different calorie intakes – 1000, 1500 and 2000. Make sure that you have worked out your daily calorie intake for the White Wine Diet as shown on pages 12-17 before you start, and remember that, once you've done this, you are also allowed two glasses of white wine and half a pint of skimmed milk in addition.

If your daily calorie intake falls in between two of these weekly meal plans, you can either adapt it by choosing different meals from the recipe section, or add extra calories by choosing foods from the list of calories on pages 191-8.

A one-week menu plan for those requiring 1000 calories per day

Day 1

Breakfast

60g pork sausage, grilled and surface fat removed
with kitchen paper
100g low-fat baked beans
1 apple

Lunch

Chicken Surprise Roll-Ups
Large Green Salad
1 banana

Dinner

Monkfish with a Trio of Vegetables
Autumn Fool

Day 2

Breakfast

1 poached egg
1 slice wholemeal toast with 15g low-fat spread

Lunch

Fruits of the Vine with Rice
1 apple

Dinner

Seaside Fish Cakes

Day 3

Breakfast

120g fresh grapefruit
45g sardines in brine spread on 1 slice wholemeal toast

Lunch

American Combination Salad

Dinner

Spicy Chicken with Dried Fruits and Colourful Peppers
25g cottage cheese
1 water biscuit
1 apple

Day 4

Breakfast

30g unsweetened muesli served with 150ml skimmed milk
60g fresh or canned pineapple in its own juice

Lunch

Welsh Potato Cakes
1 orange

Dinner

Pasta with Chicken and Vegetables

Day 5

Breakfast

25g low-fat Shreddies served with 150ml skimmed milk
1 slice wholemeal toast topped with 1 small banana

Lunch

Crispy Potato Skins with Savoury Dip

Dinner

Fish and Chickpea Curry

Day 6

Breakfast

120g strawberries served with 150ml low-fat yogurt
1 whole buttermilk pancake served with 1 teaspoon honey

Lunch

Noodles with Mushroom and Tomato Sauce

Dinner

Chicken Cassoulet
Fresh Fruit Salad with Stem Ginger

Day 7

Breakfast

60g tinned prunes
1 slice wholemeal toast topped with 60g cottage cheese
and 1 medium sliced tomato

Lunch

Tomato Upside-Down Tart
1 apple

Dinner

Spicy Lamb and Lentils
Banana and Raspberry Smoothie

A one-week menu plan for those requiring 1500 calories per day

Day 1

Breakfast

150ml tomato juice
2 slices wholemeal bread with 30g low-fat spread and
Marmite

Lunch

Fishy Soufflé Omelette
Fresh Orange Jelly

Dinner

Brown Rice Paella
Green Salad
Bread and Butter Pudding

Day 2

Breakfast

1 banana
1 slice of wholemeal bread
150ml low-fat yogurt

Lunch

Cottage Cheese Combination Salad
Rosy Poached Pears

Dinner

Pasta with Chicken and Vegetables
Surprise Nectarines with a Raspberry Sauce

Day 3

Breakfast

120g strawberries
150ml low-fat yogurt
1 whole buttermilk pancake served with 1 teaspoon honey

Lunch

Orange Roasted Fennel and Bulgar Wheat Salad
Summer Fruits

Dinner

Cheese, Onion and Potato Pie
Gooseberry Crumble
45g cheddar

Day 4

Breakfast

25g low-fat Shreddies served with 150ml skimmed milk
1 slice wholemeal toast topped with 1 small banana

Lunch

Chicken Salad
Fresh Peach with a Raspberry Coulis

Dinner

Ham in Cider
Clementine Pudding

Day 5

Breakfast

60g tinned prunes
1 slice wholemeal toast topped with 60g cottage cheese
and 1 medium sliced tomato
1 banana

Lunch

Cheesy Jacket Potato
1 apple

Dinner

Ham and Pea Risotto
Chocolate Pudding

Day 6

Breakfast

200ml fresh orange juice
1 poached egg
1 slice wholemeal toast with 15g low-fat spread
1 apple

Lunch

Mediterranean Pitta Rounds

Dinner

One-Pot Roasted Lamb
Apple Crisp Slices

Day 7

Breakfast

30g unsweetened muesli served with 150ml skimmed milk
30g very lean boiled ham served with 60g grilled fresh pineapple

Lunch

BLT Treat
1 apple
1 banana

Dinner

White Fish and Cheddar Lasagne
2 slices garlic bread made with 15g butter
Baked Apple with Currants

A one-week menu plan for those requiring 2000 calories per day

Day 1

Breakfast

100ml fresh orange juice
1 small egg, boiled or poached
1 thin slice wholemeal bread

Snack

1 apple
45g cheddar

Lunch

Sardine and Tomato Pizza
Fruity Semolina

Dinner

Indian Chickpea Salad
Cherry Cheesecake

Day 2

Breakfast

200g low-calorie baked beans
1 thin slice wholemeal bread, toasted
1 tangerine
1 apple

Snack

1 apple
45g cheddar

Lunch

Autumn Vegetable Slice
Hot and Spicy Autumn Fruits

Dinner

Chicken and Vegetable Casserole
Raisin Bread Pudding

Day 3

Breakfast

180g porridge (weight when cooked)
sweetener or salt for the porridge
90g strawberries

Snack

1 apple
45g cheddar

Lunch

Pasta and Vegetable Salad

Dinner

Sausage Casserole

Day 4

Breakfast

2 thin slices wholemeal bread
15g low-fat spread
60g smoked salmon

Snack

1 apple
45g cheddar

Lunch

Herring with Warm Potato Salad

Dinner

Spaghetti Surprise
Summer Fruit Brûlée

Day 5

Breakfast

Kedgeree
200ml fresh orange juice

Snack

1 apple
45g cheddar

Lunch

American Baked Beans

Dinner

Fish and Vegetable Pie
Pineapple and Coconut Rum Layer

Day 6

Breakfast

½ grapefruit
25g lean lightly cooked bacon, grilled
240g grilled tomatoes
1 thin slice wholemeal bread

Snack

1 apple
45g cheddar

Lunch

Tomato and Pepper Pasta with Olives
2 slices garlic bread with 15g butter

Dinner

Lamb and Potato Moussaka
Mocha Mousse

Day 7

Breakfast

120g kipper fillet
1 slice wholemeal toast

Snack

1 apple
45g cheddar

Lunch

Club Sandwich

Dinner

Garden Vegetable Soup
Ham Salad with a Difference
4 scoops low-fat ice cream

7
Cooking Low Fat –
An Essential Guide

It doesn't matter if you are on the White Wine Diet, any other diet or not even on a diet at all. If you want to keep in trim, it is a great idea to take on these few essential tips on how to cut fat out of your food.

- 1 Cal spray is a brilliant product that allows you to spray a tiny amount of oil into a pan without having to worry about adding too many calories.

- Dry-frying is an excellent way for the dieter to cook meat and poultry and, if you have a good non-stick pan, it's very straightforward. Get the pan to a medium heat before adding the food and then seal it on all sides. You can then reduce the heat and add any other ingredients.

- If you're cooking mince, add the mince to the dry pan and let it brown, stirring constantly. When cooked through, drain the fat from the mince through a colander, wipe out the pan and return the mince to continue with your recipe.

- Vegetables can be dry-fried too, as they contain their own moisture, but do be careful not to overcook them.

- Try grilling meat instead of dry-frying it. Dry the meat well using kitchen paper before eating – this will absorb any excess fat.

- Always remove any visible fat from meat and poultry before cooking it.

- Always choose the low-fat option when buying spreads, cheese or yogurt – little things like that really will make a difference to your waistline …

- Avoid eating too many calories in the evening when there is little likelihood of burning them off. What the body cannot use will be stored as fat.

- Try cooking vegetables and fish in the microwave without using oil or butter. The results can be delicious.

- Try experimenting with oil-free salad dressings. You can make delicious dressings using orange juice, lemon juice, balsamic vinegar, sushi vinegar, fat-free mayonnaise, fat-free yogurt … Go on – get creative!

8
Calorie Contents of Some Essential Foods to Help You Slim Down

Product	Calories per 30g
All-Bran	70
Almonds, fresh, shelled or ground	170
Almond paste	115
Alpen	105
Anchovy fillets or paste	45
Angel Delight	45
Apples	15
baked	10
dried	70
Apple crumble	65
Apple juice	10
Apple pie, home-made	55

The White Wine Diet

Product	Calories per 30g
Apricots, fresh, raw or stewed	5
dried	50
Artichokes, fresh or tinned	5
Asparagus, frozen	10
Aubergine	5
Avocado pear	25
Bacon, boiled, fat	95
boiled, lean	60
fried, fat	130
fried, lean	125
Bananas	20
Beans, baked	25–30
broad	10
butter	25
butter, dried	75
French, green, runner	0
green, runner, frozen	5–10
green, runner, tinned	15
haricot	25
Bean sprouts, mung	8
soya	10
Beef, boiled, silverside	85
boiled, topside	60
corned	65
roast, fat	100
roast, lean	70
Beef sausage	80
Beef stew	40
Beer, bottled, pale or brown	10
draught, pale or brown	10
strong	20
Beetroot, fresh, boiled	15
tinned	10
Blackberries, fresh, raw	10
fresh, stewed	5

Calorie Contents of Some Essential Foods

Product	Calories per 30g
frozen	10
tinned	25
Blackcurrants, same values as for blackberries	
Black pudding	70
Bounty bar	135
Bournvita, powder	105
Bovril drink	30
Bran, most natural varieties	95
Brandy, neat	75
Brazil nuts, shelled	180
Bread, white, brown or wholemeal	70
fried	160
toasted	70
Broccoli, fresh	5
frozen	10
Brussels sprouts, fresh, boiled	5
frozen	10
Butter	205
Buttermilk	10
Cabbage, boiled or raw	5
Carbonated drinks (average)	10
Carrots, fresh boiled or raw	5
Cashew nuts, salted	160
Cauliflower, boiled	5
Caviar	80
Celery, boiled	0
fresh, raw	5
Celery hearts, tinned	10
Cheddar	115
Cherries, fresh, raw	15
glacé	60
stewed	10
tinned	15
Cherry brandy	55

The White Wine Diet

Product	Calories per 30g
Cheshire cheese	105
Chestnuts, raw, shelled	50
Chicken, boiled	60
Chicory	5
Chutney, mango	15
tomato	40
Cocoa powder	135
Cod, steamed	25
Coffee, beans or instant	0
Cornflakes	100
Cottage cheese	30
Courgettes	5
Crab, boiled	35
Cranberries, fresh	5
Cream, double	130
single	60
Cream cracker	125
Cress	5
Crisps	145
Crumpets	55
toasted and buttered	210
Cucumber, raw	5
Currants	70
Custard, fresh or powdered	30
Damsons, fresh, raw or stewed	10
tinned	30
Danish Blue	105
Duck, roast	90
Edam	85
Eggs, boiled or poached	45
fried	70
scrambled	80
Endive	5
Figs, fresh	10
tinned	55

Calorie Contents of Some Essential Foods

Product	Calories per 30g
Flour, white or wholemeal	100
Gammon	60
fried	125
Garibaldi biscuit	105
Gin	65
Goose, roast, slices	90
Gooseberries, raw	10
Gorgonzola	95
Grapefruit, fresh	5
tinned	20
Greengage, raw	15
Haddock, fresh or smoked, steamed	30
fresh, fried	50
Ham, boiled, lean	60
lean and fat slices	125
Hamburger	70
Hazelnuts, shelled	110
Herring, baked	50
fried	65
Horlicks	120
Horseradish sauce	25
Hot chocolate	115
Jam, low-calorie	50
most varieties	80
Kale, boiled	10
Kipper fillets, fresh	60
Lamb chop, grilled	75
Lamb, roast, fat slices	80
roast, lean slices	55
Lard	260
Leek, boiled	5
Lemon, fresh	5
Lentils, boiled	25
Lettuce, raw	5
Lobster, fresh, boiled	35

The White Wine Diet

Product	Calories per 30g
Mackerel, fresh	55
tinned	55
Mandarin oranges, fresh	10
tinned	20
Marmalade	75
Marmite	35
Marrow, boiled	0
Martini, dry	35
Rosso, Bianco	45
Mayonnaise	110
Melon, yellow, fresh	5
Milk, condensed, skimmed	80
evaporated, tinned	45
fresh, full-fat	20
fresh, skimmed	10
Muesli	105
Mushrooms, fried	40–60
grilled, boiled	2
Mussels	25
Oatmeal porridge, boiled	15
Oil, vegetable	250
Olive oil	265
Olives	30
Omelette	55
Onion, boiled	5
fried	100
raw	5
Oranges	10
Orange juice, freshly squeezed	10
Ovaltine	110
Parmesan	120
Parsnip, boiled or raw	15
Pasta, dried or fresh	95
Peaches, dried	60
fresh	10

Calorie Contents of Some Essential Foods

Product	Calories per 30g
stewed	20
tinned	20
Peanut butter	175
Pears, fresh or stewed	10
Peas, dried	30
fresh, boiled	15
frozen	20
Peppers, red or green	5
Pilchards, tinned	55
Pineapple, fresh	10
tinned	20
Plums, fresh	10
stewed	5
tinned	20
Pork chop, grilled	155
leg roast	90
loin, lean slices	80
Potatoes, boiled	25
tinned	20
Prawns, boiled and shelled	30
Prunes, dried, stewed	20
tinned	25
Radish	5
Raspberries, fresh or frozen, raw or stewed	5
tinned	25
Red cabbage, pickled	5
Rhubarb, stewed	0
tinned	20
Rice, boiled	35
Rice Krispies	100
Ritz biscuit	150
Roquefort	90
Ryvita crispbread, white or brown	90
Salmon, fresh	55

The White Wine Diet

Product	Calories per 30g
tinned, smoked, frozen	45
Scallops, steamed	30
Sherry, dry	30
sweet	35
Shortbread	140
Shreddies	115
Shredded Wheat	115
Special K	100
Spinach, fresh, boiled	5
Spring onions	10
Stilton	95
Strawberries	5
Sugar	110
Swede, boiled	5
Sweetcorn	25
Tea	0
Tomato, fresh	5
fried	20
tinned	5
Tomato juice	5
Tomato ketchup	30
Trout, steamed	40
Turbot, steamed	30
Turkey, roast	55
Turnip, boiled or raw	5
Walnuts, shelled	150
Water biscuit	115
Watercress	5
Yogurt, low-fat	20

Index of Recipes

The White Wine Diet

The White Wine Diet